The Hands-on Guide to Clinical Pharmacology

Third Edition

The Hands-on Guide to Clinical Pharmacology

Sukhdev Chatu

Gastroenterology & General Medicine Specialist Registrar London, United Kingdom

WILEY-BLACKWELL

A John Wiley & Sons, Ltd, Publication

This edition first published 2010
© 2010 by S Chatu Previous editions: 2000, 2005

Blackwell Publishing was acquired by John Wiley & Sons in February 2007.
Blackwell's publishing program has been merged with Wiley's global Scientific,
Technical and Medical business to form Wiley-Blackwell.

Registered office:
John Wiley & Sons Ltd, The Atrium, Southern Gate, Chichester, West
Sussex, PO19 8SQ, UK

Editorial offices:
9600 Garsington Road, Oxford, OX4 2DQ, UK
The Atrium, Southern Gate, Chichester, West Sussex, PO19 8SQ, UK
111 River Street, Hoboken, NJ 07030-5774, USA

For details of our global editorial offices, for customer services and for
information about how to apply for permission to reuse the copyright material
in this book please see our website at www.wiley.com/wiley-blackwell

Library of Congress Cataloging-in-Publication Data

Chatu, Sukhdev.
   The Hands-on guide to clinical pharmacology / Sukhdev Chatu. – 3rd ed.
      p. cm.
   Rev. ed. of: Hands-on guide to clinical pharmacology / Christopher
Tofield, Alexander Milson, Sukhdev Chatu. 2nd ed. 2005.
   Includes bibliographical references and index.
   ISBN 978-1-4051-9195-1 (pbk.)
1. Clinical pharmacology–Handbooks, manuals, etc.   I. Tofield, Christopher.
Hands-on guide to clinical pharmacology.   II. Title.
   [DNLM: 1. Drug Therapy–methods–Handbooks.   2. Pharmacology,
Clinical–methods–Handbooks. QV 39 C495h 2010]
   RM301.28.C48 2010
   615′.1–dc22
                                                          2010005589

ISBN: 9781405191951

A catalogue record for this book is available from the British Library.

Typeset in 8/10pt Humanist by Aptara Inc., New Delhi, India.
Printed in Singapore by C.O.S. Printers Pte Ltd.

Contents

Preface to the third edition

Clinical pharmacology is relevant to most aspects of medicine and a basic knowledge of it is essential for those healthcare professionals involved in the clinical management of patients. With this in mind, it has become necessary to update the previous (second) edition in order to incorporate evolvements in this field.

The first edition of *Hands-on Guide to Clinical Pharmacology* was written by Alexander Milson, Christopher Tofield and me while we were still medical students (at St Bartholomew's & The Royal London Hospital School of Medicine and Dentistry). At that time, we were in need of a practical yet concise set of notes to revise clinical pharmacology. Hence, what started as a collated set of revision notes was soon expanded upon, structured and turned into the first edition.

Following the success of that original version, it soon became evident that an updated second edition was required and in demand. To the credit of all those involved in the making of that text, this success has continued to date. In this third edition, each chapter has been updated and the information expanded to include more drugs and management scenarios, as well as a new chapter on chemotherapy agents.

The purpose of this book has primarily been two-fold and remains unchanged. First, it is designed to serve as a revision aid for all students involved in the study of clinical pharmacology. Second, it is presented as a user-friendly rapid reference guide and should be of value to healthcare professionals such as medical students, doctors, pharmacists and nurses.

This book is a guide to those drugs that are most likely to be encountered on hospital wards or during a course of study. It also outlines the treatment regimens of common conditions. The most relevant and important interactions, adverse effects and contraindications have been selected. However, it is not intended as an exhaustive account of clinical pharmacology and doses have purposely been omitted. Further, more detailed information is best obtained from a local formulary (e.g. *British National Formulary*).

The aim for this book has always been accuracy while maintaining conciseness – a feature that is much valued by students and busy professionals! Certainly, this book will help you to manage pharmacology in a clinical setting and, above all, take the stress out of related exams!

S. Chatu

Acknowledgements

First and foremost, I would like to acknowledge the input of my co-authors from the first and second editions of this book, Alexander Milson and Christopher Tofield. Their contributions laid the foundation for this latest edition.

The three of us will always be grateful for the support we received, in getting the first edition off the ground, from Professor Nigel Benjamin and Professor Mark Caulfield while at St Bartholomew's & the Royal London Hospital School of Medicine and Dentistry.

I am sincerely grateful to all those colleagues who took time out of their busy schedules to check all the material and for kindly offering me their expert suggestions.

For the opportunity to update this book to its third edition I must extend my thanks to Wiley-Blackwell and also to all the staff involved in its production.

Finally, I send my heartfelt thanks to all the readers who have always been vital to the success of this venture.

Sukhdev Chatu

Abbreviations

ABG	Arterial blood gas
ACE	Angiotensin-converting enzyme
ADH	Antidiuretic hormone
ADP	Adenosine diphosphate
AF	Atrial fibrillation
ALT	Alanine transaminase
APTT	Activated partial thromboplastin time
ARB	Angiotensin-receptor blocker
5-ASA	5-aminosalicylic acid
AST	Aspartate transaminase
ATP	Adenosine triphosphate
AV	Atrioventricular
BCG	Bacillus Calmette–Guérin
BMI	Body mass index
BP	Blood pressure
BPH	Benign prostatic hyperplasia
BMI	Body mass index
cAMP	Cyclic adenosine monophosphate
CABG	Coronary artery bypass graft
CBT	Cognitive behavioural therapy
CCU	Coronary care unit
cGMP	Cyclic guanosine monophosphate
CLL	Chronic lymphoid leukaemia
CMV	Cytomegalovirus
CNS	Central nervous system
COC	Combined oral contraceptive
COMT	Catechyl-O-methyl transferase
COPD	Chronic obstructive pulmonary disease
COX	Cyclo-oxygenase
CPAP	Continuous positive airways pressure
CPR	Cardiopulmonary resuscitation
CSF	Cerebrospinal fluid
CT	Computerized tomography
CTG	Cardiotocography
CVA	Cerebrovascular accident
CXR	Chest X-ray
D_2	Dopamine$_2$
DC	Direct current
DDP-4	Dipeptidyl peptidase-4
DEXA	Dual energy X-ray absorptiometry
DMARD	Disease-modifying antirheumatic drug
DNA	Deoxyribonucleic acid
DT	Diphtheria, tetanus
DTP	Diphtheria, tetanus, pertussis
DVT	Deep vein thrombosis
EBV	Epstein–Barr virus
ECG	Electrocardiogram

ECT	Electroconvulsive therapy
EPO	Erythropoietin
FBC	Full blood count
FEV_1	Forced expiratory volume in 1 second
FSH	Follicle-stimulating hormone
5-FU	5-fluorouracil
GABA	Gamma-aminobutyric acid
G-CSF	Granulocyte-colony stimulating factor
GI	Gastrointestinal
GIP	Glucose-dependent insulinotropic polypeptide
GIST	Gastrointestinal stromal tumour
GLP-1	Glucagon-like peptide 1
GP	General practitioner
G6PD	Glucose-6-phosphate dehydrogenase
GTN	Glyceryl trinitrate
HAART	Highly active antiretroviral therapy
HACEK	**H**aemophilus (*H. parainfluenzae*, *H. aphrophilus*, *H. paraphrophilus*), **A**ctinobacillus actinomycetemcomitans (*Aggregatibacter actinomycetemcomitans*) **C**ardiobacterium hominis, **E**ikenella corrodens, **K**ingella kingae
Hb	Haemoglobin
HbA1c	Haemoglobin A1c
HBsAg	Hepatitis B surface antigen
HDL	High-density lipoprotein
Hib	*Haemophilus influenzae* type b
H_1	Histamine$_1$
H_2	Histamine$_2$
HIV	Human immunodeficiency virus
HMG-CoA	3-hydroxy 3-methylglutaryl co-enzyme A
HOCM	Hypertrophic obstructive cardiomyopathy
HPV	Human papilloma virus
HRT	Hormone replacement therapy
5-HT	5-hydroxytryptamine
ICD	Implantable cardiac defibrillator
Ig	Immunoglobulin
IHD	Ischaemic heart disease
IM	Intramuscular
INR	International normalized ratio
ISA	Intrinsic sympathomimetic activity
ISDN	Isosorbide dinitrate
ISMN	Isosorbide mononitrate
ITU	Intensive therapy unit
IUCD	Intrauterine contraceptive device
IV	Intravenous
LABA	Long-acting beta agonist
LDL	Low-density lipoprotein
LFT	Liver function test
LMWH	Low-molecular-weight heparin
LV	Left ventricular
LVEF	Left ventricular ejection fraction
LVF	Left ventricular failure

MAb	Monoclonal antibody
MAO	Monoamine oxidase
MAOI	Monoamine oxidase inhibitor
MI	Myocardial infarction
MMR	Measles, mumps, rubella
MRSA	Methicillin-resistant *Staphylococcus aureus*
NMDA	N-methyl-D-aspartate
MMSE	Mini Mental State Examination
NRT	Nicotine replacement therapy
NRTI	Nucleoside reverse transcriptase inhibitor
NRTK	Non-receptor tyrosine kinase
NSAID	Non-steroidal anti-inflammatory drug
P_{CO_2}	Partial pressure carbon dioxide
P_{O_2}	Partial pressure oxygen
PCA	Patient-controlled analgesia
PCI	Percutaneous coronary intervention
PDE_5	Phosphodiesterase type 5
PE	Pulmonary embolism
PEFR	Peak expiratory flow rate
PGE_2	Prostaglandin E_2
PID	Pelvic inflammatory disease
POP	Progestogen-only pill
PPAR	Peroxisome proliferator-activated receptor
PPI	Proton-pump inhibitor
PTH	Parathyroid hormone
PUVA	Psoralen with ultraviolet A
PSVT	Paroxysmal supraventricular tachycardia
PVD	Peripheral vascular disease
RNA	Ribonucleic acid
RTK	Receptor tyrosine kinase
SA	Sinoatrial
SC	Subcutaneous
SIADH	Syndrome of inappropriate antidiuretic hormone
SLE	Systemic lupus erythematosus
SSRI	Selective serotonin re-uptake inhibitor
STAT-C	Specifically targeted antiviral therapy for hepatitis C
SVT	Supraventricular tachycardia
T3	Triiodothyronine
T4	Thyroxine
TCA	Tricyclic antidepressant
TENS	Transcutaneous electrical nerve stimulation
TIA	Transient ischaemic attack
TIBC	Total iron-binding capacity
TKI	Tyrosine kinase inhibitor
TNF	Tumour necrosis factor
tPA	Tissue plasminogen activator
TPMT	Thiopurine methyltransferase
TSH	Thyroid-stimulating hormone
U&Es	Urea and electrolytes
UTI	Urinary tract infection
UVB	Ultraviolet B
V_2	Vasopressin$_2$

VF	Ventricular fibrillation
VLDL	Very low-density lipoprotein
V/Q	Ventilation/perfusion
VRE	Vancomycin-resistant enterococci
VT	Ventricular tachycardia
WPW	Wolff–Parkinson–White

CARDIOVASCULAR SYSTEM

The Hands-on Guide to Clinical Pharmacology, 3rd Edition. By S Chatu.
Published 2010 by Blackwell Publishing Ltd.

Furosemide
Heparin
Methyldopa
Nicorandil, nitrates (glyceryl trinitrate [GTN], isosorbide dinitrate
[ISDN], isosorbide mononitrate [ISMN])
Sildenafil, simvastatin, spironolactone
Tenecteplase
Verapamil
Warfarin

Management guidelines

ANAPHYLACTIC SHOCK
* Give 0.5 mg (0.5 ml of 1:1000) epinephrine intramuscular (IM) (given intravenous [IV] if there is no central pulse or if severely unwell) if any compromise in airway (stridor, tongue swelling), breathing (low oxygen saturations, wheeze) or circulation (hypotensive, pale, clammy).
* Most ideal site to inject IM epinephrine is the middle third of thigh on the anterolateral aspect.
* Give high-flow oxygen through face mask.
* Gain IV access.
* Give 10 mg of IV chlorpheniramine.
* Give 100–200 mg IV hydrocortisone.
* Consider salbutamol nebulizer and IV aminophylline if bronchospasm present.
* Administer IV fluids if required to maintain blood pressure (BP).
* Repeat IM epinephrine every 5 minutes if no improvement, as guided by BP, pulse and respiratory function.
* If still no improvement, consider intubation and mechanical ventilation.
* Follow-up:
    * Suggest a medic alert bracelet naming culprit allergen.
    * Identify allergen with skin prick testing and consider referral to an allergy clinic at a later stage.
    * Self-injected epinephrine may be necessary for the future.

DYSRHYTHMIAS
Bradycardia
* Look for and treat underlying cause (e.g. drugs, hypothyroidism, post MI).
* If pulse rate <40 bpm and patient symptomatic, give IV atropine up to a maximum dose of 3 mg.
* If no response, consider external, percussion or temporary venous pacing until underlying cause corrected or permanent pacemaker inserted.

Atrial fibrillation (AF)
* Look for and treat any underlying cause.
* Antiarrhythmic agents are used to restore sinus rhythm or control ventricular rate.

- Consider anticoagulation with warfarin (aspirin if warfarin contraindicated or inappropriate) to prevent thromboembolic events. The CHAD score can help in making a decision however all those with valvular heart disease should be anticoagulated
- *Paroxysmal AF*:
  - Self-terminating, usually lasts less than 48 hours.
  - If recurrent, consider warfarin and antiarrhythmic drugs (e.g. sotalol, amiodarone).
- *Persistent AF*:
  - Lasts more than 48 hours and can be converted to sinus rhythm either chemically (amiodarone, beta blocker or flecainide) or with synchronized direct current (DC) shock.
  - In cases of synchronized DC shock, administer warfarin for 1 month, then give DC shock under general anaesthetic to revert to sinus rhythm (only if no structural heart lesions are present) and continue warfarin for 1 month thereafter. If haemodynamically unstable, DC cardiovert with IV heparin or LMWH.
- *Permanent AF*:
  - To control the ventricular rate use digoxin, a rate-limiting calcium-channel blocker, beta blocker or amiodarone as monotherapy or in combination.
  - Warfarin for anticoagulation (give aspirin if warfarin is contraindicated or inappropriate) if risk of emboli is high
  - Consider pacemaker or radiofrequency ablation if all else fails.

Atrial flutter
- Look for and treat any underlying cause.
- Treat as for acute AF.
- In chronic atrial flutter, maintain on warfarin to prevent thromboembolic events and antiarrhythmic medication (e.g. sotalol, amiodarone) and consider radiofrequency ablation.

Paroxysmal supraventricular tachycardia (PSVT)
- Most terminate spontaneously, if not perform vagal manoeuvres (e.g. carotid sinus massage if no bruits, Valsalva manoeuvre), which transiently increase atrioventricular (AV) block.
- If this fails, give IV adenosine in incremental doses.
- If this fails, or adenosine is contraindicated, give IV verapamil.
- If the patient is haemodynamically compromised, give synchronized DC shock under sedation or short-acting general anaesthetic (e.g. propofol).
- Other antiarrhythmics that can be tried are beta blockers, amiodarone, flecainide, disopyramide, propafenone after seeking expert advice.
- In recurrent PSVT consider regular antiarrhythmics (commonly used drugs: beta blockers, rate-limiting calcium-channel blockers, amiodarone) or refer for radiofrequency ablation of abnormal foci.

Ventricular fibrillation (VF), pulseless ventricular tachycardia (VT)
- Protocols for the management of VF and pulseless VT are subject to constant updates. Consult current European Resuscitation Council guidelines.

Ventricular tachycardia (VT) with a pulse
- Look for and treat underlying cause and correct electrolyte imbalances.
- Give IV amiodarone or IV lidocaine.
- If this fails, consider other antiarrhythmics after expert advice (i.e. disopyramide, flecainide, procainamide, propafenone) or perform overdrive pacing.
- Proceed to synchronized DC shock if patient is symptomatic, in cases of haemodynamic compromise, or if there is no response to antiarrhythmic drugs.
- Once recovered, consider implantable cardiac defibrillator (ICD) or electrical ablation of abnormal foci or prophylaxis with a regular antiarrhythmic agent.

HEART FAILURE – ACUTE
- Sit patient up to improve oxygenation.
- Give high-flow oxygen through non-rebreathing face mask (caution in chronic obstructive pulmonary disease [COPD]).
- Consider non-invasive ventilation with positive end expiratory pressure (i.e. continuous positive airways pressure [CPAP]) if still hypoxic.
- Give IV furosemide, which initially causes venodilatation, reducing cardiac preload, and then reduces intravascular volume by diuresis.
- Give IV morphine, which relieves dyspnoea, anxiety and also cardiac preload via its venodilatory effect.
- If no improvement, consider IV GTN infusion (only if systolic BP > 100 mmHg).
- In cardiogenic shock (signified by falling BP), consider positive inotropes (dopamine, dobutamine), intra-aortic balloon pump and revascularization (percutaneous coronary intervention [PCI]), coronary artery bypass graft [CABG]) if due to an acute coronary syndrome.

HEART FAILURE – CHRONIC
- Treat any underlying cause (e.g. hypertension, valvular heart disease, ischaemic heart disease [IHD]).
- Reduce salt intake by educating patients about salt intake of common foods and alter modifiable risk factors (e.g. smoking, obesity).
- Loop diuretic (e.g. furosemide, bumetanide) for pulmonary congestion and systemic fluid overload (i.e. lower limb oedema, pleural effusions, ascites); a thiazide diuretic can be added (e.g. bendroflumethiazide or metolazone).
- Regular review and dose adjustment of diuretics required to maintain dry weight and prevent renal impairment.
- Digoxin, loop and thiazide diuretics improve symptoms only.
- All doses should be increased to target dose or maximum tolerated.
- All those with symptomatic heart failure or with asymptomatic reduced left ventricular ejection fraction (LVEF) should be started on an ACE inhibitor (e.g. ramipril).

- Beta blockers added in next, if still symptomatic.
- Aldosterone antagonist added if still symptomatic (spironolactone, eplerenone) to improve symptoms and increase survival.
- Digoxin is used first line if heart failure is associated with AF and added in sinus rhythm if still symptomatic on ACE inhibitor, beta blocker and diuretics.
- Vasodilators hydralazine and oral nitrates can be used in combination if ACE inhibitor and ARB are contraindicated or not tolerated; combination can be added to ACE inhibitor if ARB or aldosterone antagonist not tolerated.
- Start warfarin to prevent thromboembolic events if AF is present, or if there is significant cardiomegaly, left ventricle aneurysm or history of mural thrombus.
- ACE inhibitors, angiotensin-receptor blockers (ARBs), beta blockers, spironolactone, hydralazine and nitrates improve symptoms and survival in heart failure.
- Consider cardiac transplant, biventricular pacing, ICD, revascularization in IHD, valvular surgery, ventricular surgery and left ventricular assist devices (if patient meets criteria).
- Offer annual influenza and pneumococcal vaccine (only required once).
- Add aspirin if IHD also present.
- In advanced heart failure, consider palliative care.

HYPERLIPIDAEMIA

- Advise low-fat diet, substitute chicken and turkey for red meat and encourage fish, fruit, vegetables and fibre.
- Treat any underlying causes of hyperlipidaemia: hypothyroidism, chronic alcohol intake, drugs (e.g. thiazide diuretics, beta blockers).
- Medication only indicated when dietary modification fails.
- Treat for primary prevention of cardiovascular disease (MI, stroke, transient ischaemic attack [TIA], peripheral vascular disease [PVD]) in adults who have a 20% or greater 10-year risk of developing cardiovascular disease (use risk calculators).
- If cholesterol >5.5 mmol/L, start patient on a statin for primary prevention if above criteria met (use fibrate, ezetimibe, or a bile acid resin if statin not tolerated).
- Treat regardless of lipid levels if established cardiovascular disease (IHD, stroke, TIA, PVD) or diabetes present, aiming for total cholesterol of less than 4 mmol/L and low-density lipoprotein (LDL)-cholesterol of less than 2 mmol/L.
- Bile acid resins (e.g. colestyramine), nicotinic acid, ezetimibe and fibrates can also be used to decrease cholesterol levels.
- In *hypertriglyceridaemia*, fibrates (e.g. bezafibrate) are first-line therapy but nicotinic acid can also be used.
- In *mixed hyperlipidaemia* (high cholesterol and high triglycerides), statins can be used in combination with a fibrate, bile acid resin, nicotinic acid or ezetimibe.
- Omacor (omega-3-acid ethyl esters) can be used to treat hypertriglyceridaemia.

HYPERTENSION

- Alter modifiable risk factors (e.g. smoking, obesity, alcohol, salt intake).
- Rule out secondary causes of hypertension (e.g. renal disease, endocrine diseases, drugs, coarctation of the aorta).
- Indications for treatment vary but generally treat if:
    - Systolic BP sustained >160 mmHg, or
    - Diastolic BP sustained >100 mmHg.
- Treat if diastolic BP 90–99 mmHg or systolic BP 140–159 mmHg in the presence of end-organ damage (brain, heart, kidney, retina), diabetes or at high risk of IHD assessed by risk calculators.
- In diabetes and chronic kidney injury, aim for BP <130/80 mmHg.
- The following classes of antihypertensives are used in various combinations and as a general rule if under 55 years old, first line is ACE inhibitor (ARB if ACE inhibitor is contraindicated or not tolerated) and if 55 years or over, and in black patients of any age consider calcium-channel blockers and diuretics:
    1. Thiazide diuretics (e.g. bendroflumethiazide).
    2. Beta blockers (e.g. atenolol).
    3. ACE inhibitors (e.g. captopril).
    4. Calcium-channel blockers (e.g. nifedipine).
    5. ARBs (e.g. losartan).
    6. Alpha blockers (e.g. doxazosin).
    7. Centrally acting agents (e.g. methyldopa, moxonidine).

ISCHAEMIC HEART DISEASE (IHD)

Stable angina

- Alter modifiable risk factors (smoking, hypertension, hyperlipidaemia, diabetes mellitus, obesity, diet, lack of exercise).
- First-line therapy: sublingual GTN spray/tablet for acute attacks.
- Regular aspirin (if allergic or unable to tolerate aspirin, give clopidogrel).
- Maintenance therapy: beta blocker (e.g. atenolol).
- If still symptomatic, add a dihydropyridine calcium-channel blocker or a long-acting oral nitrate (isosorbide mononitrate or isosorbide dinitrate).
- If still symptomatic, give maintenance triple therapy (beta blocker, dihydropyridine calcium-channel blocker and a long-acting nitrate) + GTN for acute attacks.
- *Note*: do not give beta blockers with verapamil and exercise caution with diltiazem due to serious interactions.
- Nicorandil, a potassium-channel activator with vasodilator properties, is being increasingly used in the management of angina.
- Last resort is revascularization with percutaneous coronary intervention (PCI) or coronary bypass surgery.

Unstable angina / non-ST elevation MI / ST elevation MI

- Grouped together as acute coronary syndromes. These conditions are initially controlled medically and then investigated with a view to PCI or coronary bypass surgery.

- Sit the patient up (to ease breathing and reduce venous return to the heart).
- Give high-flow oxygen through non-rebreathing face mask (caution in COPD).
- Attach cardiac monitor and perform 12-lead electrocardiogram (ECG).
- Oral aspirin loading dose 300 mg (antiplatelet effect).
- Give oral clopidogrel loading dose 300 mg (antiplatelet activity).
- If ST elevation MI, needs urgent PCI or thrombolytic therapy if PCI not available.
- Take blood for full blood count (FBC), urea and electrolytes (U&Es), cardiac enzymes, lipids and random glucose.
- If patient is diabetic, commence on insulin sliding scale for at least 24 hours.
- Give subcutaneous (SC) low-molecular-weight heparin (LMWH) or IV heparin (to prevent infarction in acute attack) but not if having PCI.
- For pain relief, give IV morphine with IV antiemetic (e.g. metoclopramide).
- Give IV nitrates (e.g. GTN) if still symptomatic.
- If still symptomatic, start glycoprotein IIb/IIIa receptor antagonist (e.g. tirofiban – antiplatelet activity); usually started if intervention is anticipated, these drugs reduce events during and after PCI.
- If still symptomatic, consider emergency PCI or CABG surgery.
- Give IV beta blocker if not contraindicated and if haemodynamically stable (aim to maintain heart rate of 55–65 bpm to reduce myocardial work load).
- Admit to coronary care unit (CCU).

Post myocardial infarction MI
- Heparin infusion or LMWH (enoxaparin or dalteparin) may be given to maintain vessel patency (usually for 5 days).
- Some centres are using a synthetic factor X inhibitor, fondaparinux, in the treatment of acute coronary syndromes in place of heparin and LMWH.
- If pain persists, IV nitrates (e.g. GTN) and morphine can be given.
- If ST elevation persists, consider repeat thrombolysis or emergency angiogram with PCI or CABG surgery.
- Look for and treat any complications:
  - *Tachydysrhythmias*: antiarrhythmic drugs, DC shock or overdrive pacing.
  - *Bradydysrhythmias*: IV atropine, temporary pacing.
  - *LVF with pulmonary oedema*: IV furosemide followed by long-term ACE inhibitor.
  - *Cardiogenic shock*: IV dobutamine.
  - *Ventricular septal rupture/rupture of papillary muscle*: urgent surgery.
- Prevention of reinfarction:
  - Alter modifiable risk factors (smoking, obesity, hyperlipidaemia, hypertension, diabetes mellitus).
  - Daily aspirin for life, and a beta blocker (e.g. atenolol) for a minimum of 2–3 years.

- Long-term ACE inhibitor (e.g. ramipril) regardless of left ventricular (LV) function.
- If patient had a non-ST elevation MI, should continue with clopidogrel 1 year.
- Add a statin (e.g. simvastatin).
- Advise no driving for 1 month and no work for 2 months.
- Usually stay in CCU for 5 days.
- ECG stress test on day 5:
  - If satisfactory, follow up in clinic 4–6 weeks later.
  - If positive, or if ischaemic chest pain post MI, consider coronary angiogram and appropriate intervention with surgery or PCI as in- or outpatient.

THROMBOEMBOLISM
Deep vein thrombosis (DVT)
- Give IV or SC LMWH with oral warfarin.
- Alternatively use fondaparinux (synthetic factor X inhibitor) instead of heparin until adequately anticoagulated with warfarin.
- Discontinue heparin/fondaparinux when international normalized ratio (INR) reaches therapeutic range.
- Consider thrombolytic therapy (e.g. tenecteplase) in cases of large thrombi.
- Continue warfarin for a minimum of 3–6 months.
- Look for and treat underlying cause.
- Consider thrombophilia screen if no risk factors for DVT are present.

Pulmonary embolism (PE)
- Perform investigations to help confirm diagnosis (d-dimer, arterial blood gas [ABG], ECG, chest X-ray [CXR], ventilation/perfusion [V/Q] scan, computerized tomography [CT] pulmonary angiogram).
- Give high-flow oxygen through face mask.
- Give a non-steroidal anti-inflammatory drug (NSAID) for pleuritic pain.
- Give an IV heparin loading dose followed by heparin infusion or low-molecular-weight heparin or, alternatively, use fondaparinux.
- Start oral warfarin at the same time as heparin and continue warfarin for 6 months (discontinue heparin when INR reaches therapeutic range).
- Consider thrombolytic therapy (e.g. tenecteplase) if patient is haemodynamically unstable or PE suspected in cardiac arrest.
- Consider vena caval filter in recurrent PE despite adequate anticoagulation.
- Look for and treat any underlying cause.

Drug types

BETA BLOCKERS
- There are two types of beta receptors: $beta_1$ and $beta_2$.
- $Beta_1$ receptors are found in the heart.
- Most other beta receptors are $beta_2$ receptors and are found in the peripheral vasculature, kidneys, skeletal muscle and airways.

Types of beta blockers
1. *Selective* (blocking $beta_1$ receptors): atenolol, bisoprolol and metoprolol.
2. *Non-selective* (blocking both $beta_1$ and $beta_2$ receptors): nadolol, propranolol and timolol.

Indications
- Main indications:
    - Hypertension.
    - IHD.
    - Cardiac dysrhythmias.
    - Secondary prophylaxis in MI.
    - Heart failure.
- Non-selective beta blockers can further be used in:
    - Thyrotoxicosis (for symptom control).
    - Prophylaxis of migraine.
    - Glaucoma.
    - Anxiety (for prevention of palpitations, tremor and tachycardia).
    - Essential tremor.
    - Primary and secondary prophylaxis of oesophageal variceal bleeding.

Effects
- Beta blockers can cause the following effects:
    - *$Beta_1$ receptor blockade*: decreased force of myocardial contraction and decreased heart rate.
    - *$Beta_2$ receptor blockade in the kidneys*: decreased renin release and hence lowered BP.
    - *$Beta_2$ receptor blockade in skeletal muscle*: tiredness.
    - *$Beta_2$ receptor blockade in the airways*: bronchospasm.
    - *$Beta_2$ receptor blockade in blood vessels*: peripheral vasoconstriction (i.e. cold extremities).
    - Lipid-soluble beta blockers cross the blood–brain barrier and can cause sleep disturbance and nightmares (this also applies to water-soluble beta blockers, but to a lesser extent).

Note
- Selective $beta_1$ blockers may also block $beta_2$ receptors to some extent, especially in high doses.
- Beta blockers can also be either water soluble, which are excreted renally unchanged (atenolol, celiprolol, nadolol, sotalol), or lipid soluble, which are metabolized by the liver prior to excretion (metoprolol, propranolol).

- Some act as partial agonists (i.e. have intrinsic sympathomimetic activity [ISA] properties), such as celiprolol, oxprenolol and pindolol. They can simultaneously block and stimulate beta receptors. This results in less bradycardia and less peripheral vasoconstriction than with other beta blockers.
- Labetalol and carvedilol block both alpha and beta receptors.

CALCIUM-CHANNEL BLOCKERS
Types of calcium-channel blockers:
1. *Dihydropyridines*: amlodipine, felodipine, nicardipine, nifedipine, nimodipine, nisoldipine, isradipine.
2. *Phenylalkalamines*: verapamil.
3. *Benzothiazepines*: diltiazem.

Indications
- Hypertension.
- Angina.
- Supraventricular dysrhythmias (verapamil or diltiazem).

Mechanism of action
- All calcium-channel blockers act on L-type calcium channels at different sites:
    - Myocardium.
    - The conducting system of the heart.
    - Vascular smooth muscle.

Dihydropyridines
- Dihydropyridines act mainly on peripheral and coronary vasculature and are therefore used to treat angina (usually combined with a beta blocker).
- Dihydropyridines can be used alone in the treatment of hypertension or can be safely combined with a beta blocker.
- Dihydropyridines have very few cardiac effects.

Verapamil and diltiazem
- Verapamil and diltiazem act both on the heart and on peripheral blood vessels. They decrease heart rate, force of contraction and have antiarrhythmic properties. They also cause peripheral vasodilatation and dilatation of coronary arteries.
- Verapamil and diltiazem must be used with extreme caution if given with beta blockers, due to hazardous interactions such as asystole and AV-node block.

DIURETICS
Types of diuretics
1. *Thiazides*: bendroflumethiazide, benzthiazide, chlorthalidone, clopamide, cyclopenthiazide, hydrochlorothiazide, hydroflumethiazide, indapamide, metolazone, xipamide.
2. *Loop*: furosemide, bumetanide, torasemide.
3. *Potassium-sparing*: spironolactone, eplerenone, amiloride, triamterene.
4. *Carbonic anhydrase inhibitors*: acetazolamide, dorzolamide.
5. *Osmotic*: mannitol.

Indications

- Hypertension (thiazides).
- Chronic heart failure (loop diuretics, thiazides or in combination).
- Fluid overload in renal or liver disease (loop diuretics, thiazides or in combination).
- Glaucoma (acetazolamide, dorzolamide or mannitol).
- Raised intracranial pressure (mannitol).

Note

- Loop diuretics are the most effective diuretics, followed by thiazides.
- Potassium-sparing diuretics are weak and not normally used on their own. They are usually given with loop diuretics or thiazides to prevent hypokalaemia.
- Loop and thiazide diuretics act synergistically and are effective in the treatment of resistant fluid overload.

Drugs

ANGIOTENSIN-CONVERTING ENZYME (ACE) INHIBITORS

(Captopril, lisinopril, perindopril, ramipril)

Class: Angiotensin-converting enzyme (ACE) inhibitor

Indications
- Hypertension.
- Heart failure.
- Post MI in high-risk patients and if LV dysfunction.
- Diabetic nephropathy to prevent progression.

Mechanism of action
- ACE inhibitors inhibit ACE, leading to decreased synthesis of angiotensin II, a vasoconstrictor, and accumulation of bradykinin, a vasodilator, resulting in a dual antihypertensive effect. The reduction in angiotensin II leads to reduced formation of aldosterone and hence reduced sodium and water retention.
- ACE inhibitors prevent glomerular injury in the kidneys.
- ACE inhibitors are given post MI to reduce myocardial damage and prevent further coronary events as thought to:
  - Prevent atherogenesis and thrombosis in blood vessels.
  - Prevent LV hypertrophy and dysfunction.

Adverse effects
- *Common*: postural hypotension, dry cough, rash.
- *Rare*: hyperkalaemia, worsening of renal function (in those with underlying renal ischaemia or severe heart failure), angioneurotic oedema, haematological toxicity (e.g. neutropenia, agranulocytosis).

Contraindications
- Renal vascular disease (e.g. renal artery stenosis).
- Pregnancy.

Interactions
- *NSAIDs*: these increase the risk of renal impairment.
- *Potassium-sparing diuretics*: concomitant use with an ACE inhibitor increases the risk of hyperkalaemia.

Route of administration
- Oral.

Note
- Microalbuminuria is an early sign of nephropathy in diabetics. ACE inhibitors reduce the risk of further renal deterioration.
- Patients should be advised to take the first dose just before bedtime to prevent first-dose hypotension.
- ACE inhibitors improve exercise tolerance and symptoms in heart failure. They also prolong life expectancy in these patients.

Related drugs
- Cilazapril, fosinopril, imidapril, moexipril, quinapril, trandolapril.

ADENOSINE

Class: Antiarrhythmic agent

Indications
- Paroxysmal supraventricular tachycardia (PSVT).
- To differentiate between PSVT with aberrant conduction and VT.

Mechanism of action
- Adenosine acts on the sinoatrial (SA) and AV nodes by binding to adenosine receptors in the conducting tissue of the heart and by activating potassium channels. This slows conduction in the heart and causes a decrease in the heart rate.

Adverse effects
- *Common*: chest pain, bronchospasm, flushing, light-headedness, nausea (all transient, usually lasting a few seconds).
- *Rare*: severe bradycardia, transient asystole, hypotension.

Contraindications
- Asthma.
- 2nd or 3rd degree heart block (unless pacemaker *in situ*).
- Sick sinus syndrome.

Interactions
- *Dipyridamole*: enhances adenosine effects.
- *Theophylline*: inhibits the action of adenosine by blocking adenosine receptors.

Route of administration
- IV.

Note
- Prior to administration of adenosine the patient should be warned about the transient adverse effects such as chest pain, as they may cause great distress. This drug is best administrated via a large bore cannulae followed by a rapid saline flush, whilst recording a rhythm strip.
- Adenosine has a very short duration of action (about 8 seconds), therefore adverse effects are mostly short-lived. Adenosine is used in incremental amounts up to the maximum dose until the desired effect is reached.

ALPHA₁ BLOCKERS

(Doxazosin, prazosin, indoramine, terazosin, tamsulosin, alfuzosin)

Class: Alpha₁ blocker

Indications
- Hypertension.
- Benign prostatic hypertrophy (BPH).

Mechanism of action
- They inhibit alpha₁-mediated vasoconstriction, thus causing reduction in peripheral resistance with a subsequent fall in BP.
- Alpha₁ blockers relax smooth muscle in the internal urethral sphincter, resulting in increased urinary outflow in BPH.

Adverse effects
- *Common*: postural hypotension, dizziness, headache, gastrointestinal (GI) upset, fatigue.
- *Rare*: impotence, flu-like symptoms, rash.

Contraindications
- Heart failure, postural hypotension, micturition syncope.
- Caution:
  - Hepatic impairment.
  - Pregnancy.
  - Breastfeeding.

Interactions
- *Beta blockers, calcium-channel blockers, diuretics*: alpha₁ blockers enhance the hypotensive effect if used concomitantly.

Route of administration
- Oral.

Note
- Long-term therapy with doxazosin lowers plasma LDL, very low-density lipoprotein (VLDL) and triglyceride levels. It also increases high-density lipoprotein (HDL) levels and is therefore considered beneficial in patients with IHD.
- Used third line for hypertension or when other drugs are contraindicated or not tolerated.
- Doxazosin, indoramin, prazosin or terazosin can be used in the treatment of hypertension.
- Alfuzosin and tamsulosin are used in the treatment of BPH.

AMIODARONE

Class: Antiarrhythmic agent

Indications
* Supraventricular dysrhythmias.
* Ventricular dysrhythmias (including VF and pulseless VT in cardiac arrest).

Mechanism of action
* Amiodarone prolongs the refractory period in all parts of the conducting system of the heart. This decreases the speed of impulses moving through the heart.
* Amiodarone also has some beta-blocking, alpha-blocking and some weak calcium-channel-blocking properties.

Adverse effects
* *Common*: reversible corneal deposits (in long-term use), photosensitive rash.
* *Rare*: hypo- or hyperthyroidism, pulmonary fibrosis, hepatitis, neurological symptoms (e.g. tremor, ataxia), peripheral neuropathy, grey skin colour, metallic taste in the mouth, myopathy.

Contraindications
* Cardiac conduction defects (e.g. sick sinus syndrome).
* Thyroid disease.
* Pregnancy.
* Breastfeeding.
* Iodine allergy (as amiodarone contains iodine).

Interactions
* *Beta blockers*: concomitant use of amiodarone and beta blockers increases the risk of AV block, bradycardia and myocardial depression.
* *Digoxin*: amiodarone increases the plasma concentration of digoxin.
* *Diltiazem, verapamil*: concomitant use of amiodarone with diltiazem or verapamil increases the risk of AV block, bradycardia and myocardial depression.
* *Phenytoin*: amiodarone inhibits the metabolism of phenytoin.
* *Warfarin*: amiodarone enhances the effect of warfarin by inhibiting its metabolism.

Route of administration
* Oral, IV.

Note
* Thyroid function and liver function tests (LFTs) should be monitored every 6 months while on treatment with amiodarone.
* Pulmonary function tests should be performed prior to and during treatment with amiodarone in order to detect any developing pulmonary fibrosis.
* Patients should be advised to use sun block to prevent photosensitivity rash.
* Amiodarone has a half-life of about 36 days and therefore interactions can occur long after the drug has been stopped. In the emergency treatment of dysrhythmias an IV loading dose is followed by an infusion.

AMLODIPINE

Class: Calcium-channel blocker

Indications
* Hypertension.
* Prophylaxis and treatment of angina.

Mechanism of action
* Amlodipine inhibits the influx of calcium into vascular smooth muscle (and, to a lesser extent, into myocardium) by binding to the L-type calcium channels, especially in arterioles. This results in relaxation of vascular smooth muscle with a subsequent decrease in peripheral resistance and BP.
* Amlodipine dilates coronary arteries, which contributes to its antianginal effect.

Adverse effects
* *Common*: headache, flushing, ankle swelling.
* *Rare*: urinary frequency, GI disturbance, mood changes, palpitations, impotence.

Contraindications
* Breastfeeding.
* Cardiogenic shock.
* Advanced aortic stenosis.
* Unstable angina.
* Acute porphyria.

Interactions
* *Antihypertensives*: amlodipine increases the hypotensive effect.

Route of administration
* Oral.

Note
* Amlodipine can safely be used in asthmatics, for whom beta blockers are contraindicated.
* Dihydropyridine calcium-channel blockers have no antiarrhythmic properties, unlike diltiazem and verapamil.

Related drugs
* Other dihydropyridine calcium-channel blockers: felodipine, isradipine, lacidipine, lercanidipine, nicardipine, nifedipine, nimodipine, nisoldipine.

ANGIOTENSIN-RECEPTOR BLOCKERS (ARBs)

(Candesartan, eprosartan, irbesartan, losartan, olmesartan, telmisartan, valsartan)

Class: Angiotensin II-receptor blocker

Indications
- Hypertension.
- Diabetic nephropathy in type 2 diabetes mellitus to prevent progression.
- Heart failure (in combination with ACE inhibitor, or if ACE inhibitor intolerant).

Mechanism of action
- ARBs are reversible competitive antagonists at angiotensin II receptors (confusingly known as AT_1 receptors), which are found in vascular smooth muscle and in the adrenal glands. This action blocks the vasoconstrictor effects of angiotensin II, and it reduces aldosterone secretion from the adrenal cortex. These actions in turn result in an antihypertensive effect.
- ARBs do not inhibit breakdown of kinins unlike ACE inhibitors thus are rarely associated with a dry cough and angioneurotic oedema, which can make ACE inhibitors intolerable. See also Mechanism of action of ACE inhibitors.
- When the ARBs block AT_1 receptors the increased levels of angiotensin II result in stimulation of AT_2 receptors. The clinical significance of this is unknown.

Adverse effects
- *Common*: headaches, dizziness, diarrhoea.
- *Rare*: myalgia, vasculitis, hepatitis, taste disturbance, hyperkalaemia, rash, pruritus.

Contraindications
- Breastfeeding.
- Pregnancy.

Interactions
- *ACE inhibitors, ciclosporin, potassium-sparing diuretics*: concomitant use of ARBs with either of these drugs increases the risk of hyperkalaemia.

Route of administration
- Oral.

Note
- Currently only losartan and valsartan can be used to prevent renal failure in type 2 diabetes.
- Usually prescribed in clinical practice when ACE inhibitors are not tolerated or are contraindicated.

ASPIRIN

Class: Non-steroidal anti-inflammatory drug (NSAID)

Indications
- Acute coronary syndrome, acute ischaemic stroke, PVD.
- Prophylaxis of MI, ischaemic stroke, TIAs in high-risk patients.
- Mild to moderate pain and inflammation.
- In AF to prevent thromboembolic events.

Mechanism of action
- Aspirin irreversibly inhibits the cyclo-oxygenase enzymes COX-1 and COX-2. This leads to the inhibition of prostaglandin (mostly pro-inflammatory) and thromboxane (promotes clotting) synthesis leading to its effects:

1. Decrease in vascular permeability and vasodilatation (anti-inflammatory effect).

2. Decrease in sensitization of pain afferents (analgesic effect).

3. Decrease in the effect of prostaglandins on the hypothalamus (antipyretic effect).

- Platelets contain a high concentration of COX-1, which is necessary for thromboxane A_2 production. Aspirin inhibits this process and hence inhibits platelet aggregation and thrombus formation (antiplatelet effect).

Adverse effects
- *Common*: GI irritation (gastritis, duodenitis, peptic ulcer).
- *Rare*: bronchospasm, rash, thrombocytopenia, renal failure.

Contraindications
- Children under 16 years (as aspirin may cause Reye's syndrome), except when specifically indicated (e.g. juvenile arthritis).
- Active peptic ulcer or GI bleeding.
- Gout (aspirin inhibits uric acid excretion).
- Bleeding disorders (e.g. haemophilia).
- Breastfeeding.
- History of hypersensitivity.
- Intracerebral bleed.
- Uncontrolled hypertension (risk of intracerebral bleed).

Interactions
- *Selective serotonin reuptake inhibitors (SSRIs)*: concomitant use of aspirin and SSRIs increases the risk of GI bleeding.
- *Warfarin*: concomitant use of aspirin and warfarin increases the risk of bleeding.

Route of administration
- Oral, rectal.

Note
- The risk of GI irritation can be reduced by taking aspirin after food or by using the enteric-coated form.
- In high doses, aspirin can lead to salicylate intoxication (dizziness, tinnitus, deafness).

Related drugs
- Clopidogrel, dipyridamole.

ATENOLOL

Class: Beta blocker

Indications

- Hypertension.
- Angina.
- Supraventricular dysrhythmias.
- Secondary prophylaxis of MI.

Mechanism of action

- Atenolol reduces heart rate and force of myocardial contraction by acting on beta$_1$ receptors in the heart. This results in decreased workload of the heart; hence its use in angina.
- Renin production by the kidney is also reduced by atenolol, which contributes to its antihypertensive effect.
- Atenolol decreases the effects of sympathetic activity on the heart with a resulting decrease in conduction and in action potential initiation; hence its use as an antiarrhythmic.

Adverse effects

- *Common*: lethargy (usually ceases after long-term use), bradycardia and AV block, hypotension, cold peripheries.
- *Rare*: bronchospasm, worsened or precipitated heart failure, nightmares, impotence.

Contraindications

- Asthma.
- Uncontrolled heart failure (including cardiogenic shock).
- Cardiac conduction defects (e.g. 2nd and 3rd degree heart block).
- Bradycardia.
- COPD.
- Severe PVD.
- Hypotension.
- Phaeochromocytoma (can use with alpha blocker).

Interactions

- *Diltiazem*: concomitant use of diltiazem and atenolol increases the risk of bradycardia and AV block.
- *Verapamil*: the risk of heart failure, severe hypotension and asystole is increased if atenolol is given with verapamil.

Route of administration

- Oral, IV.

Note

- Atenolol is selective for beta$_1$ receptors, but at high doses it can also block beta$_2$ receptors, thus causing bronchospasm.
- Abrupt withdrawal of atenolol may worsen angina.
- Beta blockers may mask the symptoms of hypoglycaemia caused by oral hypoglycaemics or insulin.
- Bisoprolol, carvedilol or metoprolol can be used in the treatment of chronic heart failure.

Related drugs

- Bisoprolol, carvedilol, celiprolol, esmolol, labetalol, metoprolol, nadolol, oxprenolol, pindolol, propranolol, sotalol, timolol.

ATROPINE

Class: Muscarinic antagonist

Indications
- Cardiac arrest (asystole, pulseless electrical activity if rate <60 bpm).
- Bradycardia.
- Organophosphorus poisoning.
- For paralysis of the ciliary muscle (allowing measurement of the refractive error in children).
- Anterior uveitis.

Mechanism of action
- Atropine decreases the activity of the parasympathetic nervous system by blocking the action of acetylcholine on muscarinic receptors. This leads to pupillary dilatation, bronchodilatation, increase in heart rate and decreased secretions from sweat, salivary and bronchial glands.
- Atropine also reduces gut motility and bronchial secretions.

Adverse effects
- *Common*: antimuscarinic effects (e.g. dry mouth, blurred vision, constipation, dilated pupils).
- *Rare*: confusion (especially in the elderly), palpitations, irritation of the eye (when given as eye drops), acute urinary retention.

Contraindications
- BPH.
- Closed-angle glaucoma.
- Paralytic ileus.
- Myasthenia gravis.
- Pyloric stenosis.

Interactions
- *Tricyclic antidepressants (TCAs), monoamine oxidase inhibitors (MAOIs) and antihistamines*: increased risk of antimuscarinic side-effects.

Route of administration
- IV (bradycardia, cardiac arrest), IM (organophosphorus poisoning), eye drops.

Note
- Atropine can be used to reverse the adverse effects of neostigmine (e.g. excessive bradycardia). In this case it is given IV.
- When used in anterior uveitis, aim of treatment is to prevent complications.
- Occasionally, atropine is given with anaesthetics such as propofol, halothane and suxamethonium to prevent bradycardia and hypotension during general anaesthesia.
- Atropine is also used to decrease salivary and bronchial secretions that are increased during intubation prior to surgery.

BENDROFLUMETHIAZIDE

Class: Thiazide diuretic

Indications
- Hypertension.
- Chronic heart failure.
- Oedema secondary to liver disease, nephrotic syndrome or low-protein diet.
- Prophylaxis of calcium-containing renal stones.

Mechanism of action
- Bendroflumethiazide acts on the proximal part of the distal tubule in the nephron where it inhibits Na^+ and Cl^- reabsorption. This leads to increased excretion of Na^+, Cl^- and water, which stimulates potassium excretion further down in the distal tubule. All these events lead to hypokalaemia, hyponatraemia and a decrease in intravascular volume.
- Reduced intravascular volume causes an initial decrease in cardiac output (hence initial antihypertensive effect), but a reduction in peripheral resistance is responsible for lowering BP in the long term.

Adverse effects
- *Common*: hypokalaemia, hyponatraemia, dehydration, postural hypotension.
- *Rare*: impotence, hyperuricaemia, hyperglycaemia, hyperlipidaemia, hypercalcaemia, thrombocytopenia, photosensitivity, acute pancreatitis.

Contraindications
- Hypokalaemia, hyponatraemia, hypercalcaemia.
- Gout.
- Addison's disease.

Interactions
- *Digoxin*: hypokalaemia caused by bendroflumethiazide potentiates the effects of digoxin.
- *Lithium*: bendroflumethiazide increases the plasma concentration of lithium.

Route of administration
- Oral.

Note
- Low doses of bendroflumethiazide cause minimal biochemical disturbance and are fully effective at lowering BP. Higher doses do not decrease BP any further, but make biochemical adverse effects more likely.
- Prolonged use at high doses may lead to hypokalaemia, which may cause cardiac dysrhythmias (hence potassium levels must be monitored). If high doses are prescribed, it is recommended to combine bendroflumethiazide with either potassium supplements, a potassium-sparing diuretic (e.g. amiloride) or an ACE inhibitor.

Related drugs
- Chlorthalidone, cyclopenthiazide, hydrochlorothiazide, indapamide, metolazone, xipamide.

CARDIOVASCULAR SYSTEM

BEZAFIBRATE

Class: Fibrate

Indications
- Hyperlipidaemia.

Mechanism of action
- Bezafibrate reduces triglyceride levels by stimulating the enzyme lipoprotein lipase, which converts triglycerides into fatty acids and glycerol.
- Bezafibrate also reduces cholesterol levels (to a lesser extent than triglycerides) by reducing cholesterol production in the liver. It decreases circulating LDL levels and also increases the levels of beneficial HDL.

Adverse effects
- *Common*: nausea, abdominal discomfort, headache.
- *Rare*: myositis syndrome (muscle pain, stiffness, weakness), impotence, rash, pruritus, gallstones.

Contraindications
- Hepatic impairment.
- Pregnancy and breastfeeding.
- Nephrotic syndrome.
- Gallbladder disease.
- Primary biliary cirrhosis.

Interactions
- *Statins*: concomitant use of bezafibrate and statins increases the risk of myositis syndrome.
- *Warfarin*: bezafibrate potentiates the anticoagulant effect of warfarin by displacing it from plasma protein binding sites.

Route of administration
- Oral.

Note
- Drug treatment of hyperlipidaemia is recommended when patients fail to respond to dietary measures.
- It has been shown that fibrates are less effective than statins in the prevention of cardiovascular events (e.g. MI, stroke).

Related drugs
- Ciprofibrate, fenofibrate, gemfibrozil.

CLOPIDOGREL

Class: Antiplatelet drug

Indications
- Prevention of vascular events after ischaemic stroke, after MI and in PVD.
- Acute coronary syndrome.
- Post coronary artery stent (1 year for drug eluted, up to 3 months for bare metal stent).

Mechanism of action
- Clopidogrel irreversibly modifies adenosine diphosphate (ADP) receptors on platelets and thus prevents ADP from binding to them. This prevents activation of glycoprotein GpIIb/IIIa complex and therefore prevents platelet aggregation.
- Platelets exposed to clopidogrel are affected for the rest of their lifespan, which is 8–10 days.

Adverse effects
- *Common*: GI symptoms, rash.
- *Rare*: bleeding (GI tract, intracranial), neutropenia, thrombotic thrombocytopenic purpura, hepatic impairment.

Contraindications
- Active bleeding.
- Breastfeeding.
- Intracranial bleed.

Interactions
- Anticoagulants or *other antiplatelet drugs*: increase the risk of bleeding.
- *NSAIDs:* increase the risk of bleeding.

Route of administration
- Oral.

Note
- Clopidogrel is used when aspirin is contraindicated or not tolerated.
- Clopidogrel can be combined with aspirin in the treatment of acute coronary syndromes for a more effective antiplatelet effect.

Related drugs
- Other antiplatelet drugs: abciximab, aspirin, dipyridamole, eptifibatide, tirofiban.

DIGOXIN

Class: Cardiac glycoside

Indications
* Supraventricular dysrhythmias.
* Chronic heart failure.

Mechanism of action
* Increases the force of myocardial contraction by inhibiting the Na^+/K^+ adenosine triphosphate (ATP) pump in the heart. This increases intracellular Na^+ concentration, which in turn inhibits the Na^+/Ca^{2+} exchanger and hence the amount of calcium pumped out of the cell. These events lead to increased intracellular calcium in myocardial cells, which increases myocardial contraction.
* Digoxin slows the heart rate by increasing vagal activity. It also slows conduction through the AV node (hence its use in dysrhythmias).

Adverse effects
* *Common*: nausea, vomiting, anorexia, diarrhoea, arrhythmias.
* *Rare*: gynaecomastia in chronic use, confusion, hallucinations, yellow vision, thrombocytopenia.

Contraindications
* 2nd or 3rd degree heart block.
* Hypertrophic obstructive cardiomyopathy (HOCM).
* AV accessory pathway, e.g. Wolff–Parkinson–White (WPW) syndrome.
* VT or VF.

Interactions
* *Amiodarone, propafenone, quinidine*: these antiarrhythmic drugs increase the risk of digoxin toxicity.
* *Diltiazem, nicardipine, verapamil*: increase the risk of digoxin toxicity.

Route of administration
* Oral, IV (for emergency loading dose).

Note
* In chronic heart failure, digoxin does not reduce mortality but improves symptoms and reduces the frequency of hospital admissions.
* For treatment of dysrhythmias, a loading dose is given IV or orally but this is not required in the treatment of chronic heart failure.
* Digoxin has a narrow therapeutic window and therefore requires therapeutic drug monitoring.
* The risk of digoxin toxicity is greater in hypokalaemia. Patients receiving digoxin and potassium-losing diuretics may therefore require potassium supplements or a potassium-sparing diuretic.
* Hypomagnesaemia, hypercalcaemia and hypothyroidism also increase the risk of digoxin toxicity.
* Digoxin can cause ST depression and T wave changes on the ECG, which do not indicate toxicity.

Related drugs
* Digitoxin.

DILTIAZEM

Class: Calcium-channel blocker

Indications
- Prophylaxis and treatment of angina.
- Hypertension.
- Paroxysmal supraventricular dysrhythmias (treatment and prophylaxis).
- Rate control in AF and atrial flutter.

Mechanism of action
- Diltiazem inhibits the influx of calcium into vascular smooth muscle and myocardium by binding to the L-type calcium channels. This results in:

1. Relaxation of vascular smooth muscle with subsequent decrease in peripheral resistance and BP.

2. Decreased myocardial contractility.

3. Slowed conduction at the AV node and prolonged refractory period (hence its use as an antiarrhythmic).

- Reduction in afterload, myocardial contractility and heart rate lead to reduced oxygen consumption, thereby relieving angina.

Adverse effects
- *Common*: headache, dizziness, hypotension, bradycardia, ankle swelling, constipation.
- *Rare*: lethargy, rash, AV block.

Contraindications
- Severe bradycardia.
- 2nd and 3rd degree heart block (unless pacemaker).
- Sick sinus syndrome, WPW syndrome, accessory pathways.
- Heart failure.
- Pregnancy and breastfeeding.
- Acute porphyria.

Interactions
- *Antiarrhythmics*: diltiazem may potentiate the myocardial depression caused by other antiarrhythmic drugs.
- *Beta blockers*: these increase the risk of AV block and bradycardia if given with diltiazem.
- *Digoxin*: diltiazem increases the plasma concentration of digoxin.
- *Theophylline*: diltiazem enhances the effects of theophylline.

Route of administration
- Oral.

Note
- Diltiazem can be used in patients with coronary artery spasm (Prinzmetal's angina).
- Diltiazem has the fewest adverse effects of all calcium-channel blockers.
- It has a short half-life due to extensive first-pass metabolism.
- Topical diltiazem can be used to treat chronic anal fissure.

Related drugs
- Verapamil.

DOBUTAMINE

Class: Inotropic sympathomimetic.

Indications
- Inotropic support in the following:
  - Cardiogenic shock.
  - Cardiac surgery.
  - Septic shock.
- Pharmacological cardiac stress testing.

Mechanism of action
- Dobutamine stimulates beta$_1$ receptors in the heart. This results in increased cardiac contractility.
- Unlike dopamine, dobutamine does not cause release of norepinephrine.

Adverse effects
- *Common*: tachycardia (dobutamine has a lesser tendency to cause tachycardia than dopamine), temporary premature ventricular beats, temporary rise in BP.
- *Rare*: cardiac dysrhythmias, shortness of breath.

Contraindications
- None.

Interactions
- *Beta blockers*: severe hypertension may occur.

Route of administration
- IV.

Note
- Dobutamine does not reduce renal perfusion and for this reason is preferred to beta agonists in the treatment of shock.
- Other vasoconstrictor agents used in the intensive therapy unit (ITU) setting to correct hypotension are the alpha$_1$ receptor agonists: ephedrine, metaraminol, phenylephrine.

Related drugs
- Dopamine, dopexamine.

DOPAMINE

Class: Inotropic sympathomimetic.

Indications

- Cardiogenic shock following MI.
- Hypotension following cardiac surgery.
- Initiation of diuresis in chronic heart failure.

Mechanism of action

- The actions of dopamine are dose dependent.
- In low doses (<5 μg/kg/min), dopamine acts on dopamine receptors resulting in renal, coronary and mesenteric vasodilatation. This improves perfusion in those areas.
- In moderate doses (5–20 μg/kg/min), dopamine increases cardiac contractility and causes tachycardia by acting on cardiac beta$_1$ adrenoceptors.
- In high doses (>20 μg/kg/min), dopamine causes vasoconstriction by acting on alpha adrenoceptors.

Adverse effects

- *Common:*
  - Low doses: nausea, vomiting.
  - Moderate to high doses: tachycardia, ventricular ectopic beats, peripheral vasoconstriction, hypotension or hypertension.

Contraindications

- Untreated tachydysrhythmias.
- Phaeochromocytoma.

Interactions

- *MAOIs*: dopamine can cause a hypertensive crisis if given with MAOIs.

Route of administration

- IV.

Note

- Moderate and high doses of dopamine must be administered through a central venous line.
- BP, heart rate and urine output must be monitored during treatment.
- Dopamine should not be infused into alkaline solutions as this would render it inactive.
- Extravasation of dopamine can cause skin necrosis. If this occurs, phentolamine should be infiltrated into the ischaemic area because this neutralizes the dopamine.

Related drugs

- Dobutamine, dopexamine.

EPINEPHRINE (ADRENALINE)

Class: Sympathomimetic agent

Indications
- Anaphylaxis.
- Cardiac arrest.
- Prolongation of the effects of local anaesthetics.
- Open-angle glaucoma.
- Severe asthma and croup.
- Endoscopic therapy, e.g. bleeding peptic ulcer.

Mechanism of action
- Epinephrine has various effects due to stimulation of the sympathetic nervous system. It is a potent alpha and beta receptor agonist. It is more beta$_2$ selective, but does not distinguish between alpha$_1$ and alpha$_2$ receptors.
- Beta$_1$ receptor stimulation increases the heart rate and force of myocardial contraction. Beta$_2$ receptor stimulation results in vasodilatation, bronchodilatation and uterine relaxation.
- Alpha receptor stimulation causes vasoconstriction, which prolongs the action of local anaesthetics by preventing their spread from the site of application.
- In anaphylactic shock, epinephrine raises BP and causes bronchodilatation.
- Epinephrine is thought to decrease the production of aqueous humour and increase its outflow from the anterior chamber of the eye, hence its use in glaucoma.
- In asthma and croup, epinephrine reduces bronchial muscle spasm and decreases airway swelling, respectively.

Adverse effects
- *Common*: anxiety, restlessness, tremor, tachycardia, hypertension.
- *Rare*: cardiac dysrhythmias, cerebral haemorrhage, pulmonary oedema (all in overdose).

Contraindications
- Closed-angle glaucoma.

Interactions
- *Beta blockers*: can cause severe hypertension if given with epinephrine.
- *Tricyclic antidepressants*: increase the risk of cardiac dysrhythmias and hypertension if given with epinephrine (local anaesthetics with adrenaline are safe).

Route of administration
- IM (anaphylactic shock), IV (cardiac arrest), SC (with local anaesthetics), inhalation (asthma, croup), eye drops (open-angle glaucoma).

Note
- Epinephrine is frequently administered with local anaesthetics (e.g. lidocaine) except in the fingers, toes and penis where prolonged vasoconstriction may result in gangrene.
- In cardiac arrest, epinephrine can be given through an endotracheal tube if IV access is unobtainable. In this case the dose should be doubled.

EZETIMIBE

Class: Cholesterol-absorption inhibitor

Indications
- Hypercholesterolaemia.

Mechanism of action
- Reduces cholesterol absorption from the intestine, which leads to reduced cholesterol delivery to the liver. This causes increased hepatic LDL-receptor activity, thereby increasing clearance of plasma LDL cholesterol.
- Ezetimibe is absorbed form the intestine and is transferred to the liver via the portal circulation and is excreted back into the duodenum with bile. This repeated enterohepatic metabolism accounts for its long half-life of about 22 hours.

Adverse effects
- *Common*: GI symptoms, headache.
- *Rare*: myalgia, myopathy, rhabdomyolysis, hepatitis, gallstones, cholecystitis.

Contraindications
- Nil.

Interactions
- *Ciclosporin*: plasma concentration of both drugs is increased.
- *Fibrates*: increased risk of gallstones if used with ezetimibe.

Route of administration
- Oral.

Note
- Usually used in conjunction with a statin due to their additive effect but can be used as monotherapy.
- Ezetimibe also causes a reduction in triglyceride levels.

FUROSEMIDE (FRUSEMIDE)

Class: Loop diuretic

Indications
- Acute and chronic heart failure.
- Fluid overload (i.e. acute or chronic kidney injury, ascites in cirrhosis).
- Hypercalcaemia.

Mechanism of action
- Furosemide inhibits reabsorption of Na^+, K^+, Cl^-, H^+ and water in the ascending limb of the loop of Henle in the kidneys by inhibiting the $Na^+/K^+/2Cl^-$ pump at this site. This leads to increased salt, water and potassium loss and can lead to side-effects of hyponatraemia, hypokalaemia and hypochloraemia.
- Furosemide further decreases preload by causing venodilatation. This reduces ventricular filling pressures in the heart thereby reducing myocardial work load. This effect occurs before the diuretic response.

Adverse effects
- *Common*: hypovolaemia, hypokalaemia, hyponatraemia, hyperuricaemia and gout.
- *Rare*: bone marrow suppression, GI disturbance, reversible deafness (only in high doses or in patients with renal failure), hypocalcaemia, acute pancreatitis.

Contraindications
- Renal failure with anuria.

Interactions
- *Antibacterials*: furosemide increases the risk of ototoxicity associated with aminoglycosides and vancomycin.
- *Digoxin*: furosemide-induced hypokalaemia enhances the effects of digoxin, thus increasing the risk of digoxin-induced dysrhythmias.
- *Lithium*: furosemide decreases lithium excretion, leading to an increased risk of lithium toxicity.
- *NSAIDs*: concomitant use increases the risk of nephrotoxicity and reduces response of loop diuretics.

Route of administration
- Oral, IM, IV.

Note
- Furosemide causes potassium loss. A potassium-sparing diuretic (e.g. amiloride), potassium supplements or an ACE inhibitor should be prescribed with it.
- Relief of breathlessness in acute pulmonary oedema results from venodilatation and preload reduction before diuresis.
- Loop diuretics are more effective than thiazide diuretics.
- In renal impairment, higher doses of diuretics are required as there is reduced luminal excretion of the drug, reducing its effects.

Related drugs
- Bumetanide, torasemide.

HEPARIN

Class: Anticoagulant

Indications
- Prophylaxis and treatment of DVT and PE.
- Acute coronary syndrome.
- Acute occlusion of peripheral arteries.
- Extracorporeal circuits (e.g. haemodialysis, cardiopulmonary bypass).

Mechanism of action
- Heparin potentiates the action of antithrombin III, which inactivates thrombin and other clotting factors (especially Xa) involved in the clotting pathway. This inhibits thrombus formation.
- Heparin has an antiplatelet effect by binding to and inhibiting von Willebrand factor.

Adverse effects
- *Common*: haemorrhage.
- *Rare*: osteoporosis or alopecia with long-term use, skin necrosis, rash, anaphylaxis, heparin-induced thrombocytopenia, hyperkalaemia.

Contraindications
- Haemorrhage.
- Haemophilia/thrombocytopenia.
- Active peptic ulceration.
- Following major trauma.
- Recent haemorrhagic stroke or recent surgery.
- Severe hypertension.
- Severe liver disease.
- Renal impairment (caution with LMWH).

Interactions
- *Aspirin and clopidogrel*: both increase the risk of haemorrhage if given with heparin.
- *Glyceryl trinitrate*: a GTN infusion increases the excretion of heparin.

Route of administration
- IV, SC.

Note
- Two types of heparin are available: unfractionated heparin and LMWH. They are both of equal efficacy, but LMWH has a longer duration of action (e.g. dalteparin).
- LMWH is preferred because it can be given SC and avoids the need for activated partial thromboplastin time (APTT) monitoring.
- Heparin-induced thrombocytopenia usually occurs day 5–10 after treatment and is characterized by a reduction in platelet count, thrombosis and a skin reaction. Heparin must be stopped and an alternative anticoagulant used.

Related drugs
- Other LMWHs: bemiparin, dalteparin, enoxaparin, tinzaparin.

METHYLDOPA

Class: Centrally acting antihypertensive agent

Indications
* Hypertension.

Mechanism of action
* Methyldopa is converted to its active component, alpha-methylnorepinephrine, within adrenergic nerve endings. This compound stimulates $alpha_2$ adrenoceptors of the vasomotor centre in the medulla, causing reduced sympathetic outflow. Subsequently, this leads to vasodilatation and a fall in BP.

Adverse effects
* *Common*: drowsiness, headache, postural hypotension, depression, impotence.
* *Rare*: haemolytic anaemia, diarrhoea, nasal congestion, hepatitis, gynaecomastia.

Contraindications
* Depression.
* Active liver disease.
* Acute porphyria.
* Phaeochromocytoma.

Interactions
* *Anaesthetics*: these enhance the hypotensive effect of methyldopa.
* *Antidepressants*: these enhance the hypotensive effect of methyldopa.
* *Lithium*: concomitant use of methyldopa and lithium may cause neurotoxicity.

Route of administration
* Oral, IV.

Note
* Methyldopa is commonly prescribed for hypertension in pregnancy. It crosses the placenta and appears in breast milk but has no adverse effects on the fetus.
* Treatment with methyldopa may result in a positive direct Coombs test.

Related drugs
* Clonidine, moxonidine.

NICORANDIL

Class: Potassium-channel activator

Indications
- Prevention and treatment of stable angina.

Mechanism of action
- Nicorandil's actions include both nitrate-like effects and activation of ATP-sensitive potassium channels in vascular smooth muscle. This leads to vasodilatation in coronary, arterial and venous systems, which in turn reduces preload, afterload and myocardial oxygen consumption.
- Nicorandil has no significant effects on myocardial contractility.

Adverse effects
- *Common*: headache, nausea, vomiting, dizziness, facial flushing.
- *Rare*: angina, palpitations, GI tract and anal ulceration, myalgia, angioedema, bronchitis, dyspnoea.

Contraindications
- Cardiogenic shock.
- Hypotension.
- LVF.
- Breastfeeding.

Interactions
- *MAOIs*: enhance the hypotensive effect.
- *Sildenafil, tadalafil, vardenafil*: enhance the hypotensive effect.

Route of administration
- Oral.

Note
- Headaches usually diminish with continued use.
- Nicorandil has been shown to reduce the incidence of VTs/PSVTs and myocardial ischaemia in patients already on maximum conventional antianginal therapy. This effect is believed to be due to nicorandil mimicking the natural process of ischaemic preconditioning, whereby the heart's inbuilt mechanism makes it more and more resistant to ischaemic episodes.
- Nicorandil is currently the only potassium-channel activator in use.
- Nicorandil should be considered as a possible cause in patients who present with symptoms of perianal or GI ulceration. They will only respond to treatment withdrawal.

NITRATES

(Glyceryl trinitrate, isosorbide mononitrate, isosorbide dinitrate)

Class: Organic nitrates

Indications
- Angina and acute coronary syndromes.
- Heart failure (acute LVF, chronic heart failure).
- Malignant hypertension.
- Anal fissure (applied as GTN ointment).

Mechanism of action
- Nitrates are metabolized into nitric oxide within vascular smooth muscle cells. This compound causes relaxation of vascular smooth muscle through activation of guanylyl cyclase. As a result, coronary arteries and systemic veins vasodilate, with ensuing decrease in preload and improved oxygen supply to the myocardium, which reduces LV work load.
- Nitrates also reduce afterload to some extent. This is useful in the treatment of heart failure.

Adverse effects
- *Common*: headache, dizziness, postural hypotension, flushing, tachycardia.

Contraindications
- Hypotension or hypovolaemia.
- Aortic or mitral stenosis.
- Constrictive pericarditis.
- Cardiac tamponade.
- HOCM.
- Closed-angle glaucoma
- Taking sildenafil, tadalafil, or vardenafil.

Interactions
- *Sildenafil, tadalafil, vardenafil*: enhance the hypotensive effect of nitrates.

Route of administration
- Sublingual, skin patch or skin ointment (all for angina), IV (for unstable angina, acute heart failure, malignant hypertension), oral (for angina, heart failure).

Note
- Sublingual GTN or a GTN skin patch can be used prophylactically before exercise to prevent angina.
- Properties of isosorbide dinitrate and isosorbide mononitrate are similar to those of GTN but they can be taken orally and have a longer duration of action.
- Tolerance to long-acting nitrates (ISDN and ISMN) develops after as little as 24 hours of continued administration. Their effects thus become progressively weaker. This can be minimized by allowing drug-free periods of 8 hours.

SILDENAFIL

Class: Phosphodiesterase type 5 (PDE$_5$) inhibitor

Indications
* Male erectile dysfunction.
* Primary pulmonary hypertension.

Mechanism of action
* Penile erection in a healthy male involves nitric oxide release within the corpus cavernosum in response to sexual stimulation. Nitric oxide increases the levels of cyclic guanosine monophosphate (cGMP) through activation of guanylate cyclase. This leads to relaxation of smooth muscle within the corpus cavernosum and allows influx of blood.
* The role of phosphodiesterase type 5 (PDE$_5$) is to degrade cGMP within the corpus cavernosum. Sildenafil selectively inhibits PDE$_5$, leading to increased cGMP resulting in prolonged relaxation of smooth muscle in the penis and maintenance of an erection in response to sexual stimulation.
* Sildenafil leads to vasodilatation of pulmonary blood vessels, hence is used in primary pulmonary hypertension.

Adverse effects
* *Common*: headache, flushing, nasal congestion, dyspepsia.
* *Rare*: cardiovascular events (acute coronary syndromes, arrhythmias), priapism, dizziness, hypersensitivity reactions, visual disturbance.

Contraindications
* Concomitant use of nitrates.
* Hypotension (systolic <90 mmHg).
* Recent stroke.
* MI and unstable angina.
* Hereditary degenerative disorders of the retina.

Interactions
* *Nicorandil*: concomitant use may lead to profound hypotension.
* *Nitrates*: concomitant use may lead to profound hypotension.
* *Ritonavir*: this raises the plasma concentration of sildenafil.

Route of administration
* Oral.

Note
* At recommended doses, sildenafil will not produce an erection without sexual stimulation.
* Important to illicit cause of impotence before prescribing medication, e.g. vascular, endocrine, neurological, psychological or drug induced.
* After taking a dose of sildenafil, the patient has a 4-hour window to engage in sexual intercourse. Other PDE$_5$ inhibitors have a longer duration of action (16 hours for vardenafil, 3 days for tadalafil).
* If prolonged erection (priapism >4 hours) urgent treatment is required to prevent irreversible damage with penile aspiration of blood, lavage, medical or surgical treatment.

Related drugs
* Tadalafil, vardenafil.

SIMVASTATIN

Class: HMG CoA reductase inhibitor

Indications
- Hypercholesterolaemia.
- Mixed hyperlipidaemia.

Mechanism of action
- Statins mainly target hepatocytes in the liver and reversibly inhibit HMG CoA reductase, the rate-limiting enzyme in cholesterol synthesis by the liver. The liver responds by increasing expression of LDL receptors, which increases LDL uptake from the plasma. These actions reduce plasma LDL cholesterol and therefore total cholesterol.
- Simvastatin causes a small decrease in the plasma concentration of triglycerides.
- Statins also have other non-lipid effects that provide benefit apart from lipid reduction, e.g. improve endothelial function, plaque stabilization, anti-inflammatory effects.

Adverse effects
- *Common*: headache, muscle cramps, flatulence.
- *Rare*: reversible myositis, GI disturbance (diarrhoea, abdominal pain), rash, alopecia, altered LFTs, hepatitis, acute pancreatitis.

Contraindications
- Acute liver disease or unexplained persistent abnormal LFTs.
- Pregnancy and breastfeeding.
- Acute porphyria.

Interactions
- *Ciclosporin, clarithromycin, erythromycin*: increase risk of myositis if given with simvastatin.
- *Fibrates*: increase the risk of myositis if given with simvastatin.
- *Itraconazole and ketoconazole*: increase the risk of myopathy if given with simvastatin.
- *Warfarin*: simvastatin enhances the effect of warfarin.

Route of administration
- Oral.

Note
- Simvastatin has been shown to be effective in reducing cardiovascular events and mortality in patients with known, or at high risk of, cardiovascular disease.
- Simvastatin should only be prescribed if the patient has not responded sufficiently to diet modification and after secondary causes of hyperlipidaemia have been ruled out (e.g. hypothyroidism, chronic alcohol abuse).
- LFTs should be carried out before, and 3 months after, starting therapy and yearly after unless clinically indicated.
- Statins should be taken at night as cholesterol is synthesized mainly during sleep (atorvastatin can be taken at any time).
- The patient should be advised to immediately report unexplained muscle pain, tenderness or weakness.

Related drugs
- Atorvastatin, fluvastatin, pravastatin, rosuvastatin.

SPIRONOLACTONE

Class: Aldosterone antagonist

Indications
- Chronic heart failure.
- Conn's syndrome.
- Treatment of ascites in cirrhosis.
- Hypertension.

Mechanism of action
- Aldosterone causes sodium and therefore fluid retention and potassium excretion. Spironolactone is a competitive antagonist of aldosterone and acts on the distal tubule in the kidneys to inhibit its effects. This leads to a diuretic action with sodium excretion and potassium retention.
- There are high levels of aldosterone in heart failure thought to cause myocardial fibrosis, endothelial dysfunction and arrhythmias; spironolactone inhibits these processes by acting on the myocardium.

Adverse effects
- *Common*: hyperkalaemia, gynaecomastia, male sexual dysfunction, menstrual irregularities.
- *Rare*: hepatotoxicity, osteomalacia, headache, confusion, rashes.

Contraindications
- Hyperkalaemia.
- Addison's disease.

Interactions
- *ACE inhibitors, ARBs, potassium supplements*: these drugs increase the risk of hyperkalaemia if used concomitantly with spironolactone.

Route of administration
- Oral.

Note
- Monitor renal function and serum potassium during treatment and if hyperkalaemia develops the dose should be halved or treatment stopped.
- Low doses are used in chronic heart failure but in ascites due to cirrhosis higher doses are usually required.

Related drugs
- Eplerenone.

TENECTEPLASE

Class: Fibrinolytic agent

Indications
* Acute myocardial infarction (ST elevation MI).
* Acute PE with haemodynamic compromise.
* Acute ischaemic stroke (only alteplase licensed).

Mechanism of action
* Tenecteplase is a tissue plasminogen activator (tPA).
* It binds to circulating plasminogen in the blood and forms an activator complex that converts plasminogen to plasmin. Plasmin then lyses the fibrin within the thrombus, thus dissolving it.

Adverse effects
* *Common*: bleeding from vascular puncture sites, GI bleed from occult peptic ulcers, nausea, vomiting, hypotension.
* *Rare*: intracerebral haemorrhage, allergic reaction.

Contraindications
* Recent haemorrhage.
* Bleeding disorders.
* Recent trauma or surgery.
* Aortic dissection.
* Severe hepatic impairment.
* Acute pancreatitis.
* Coma.
* Severe hypertension.
* Suspected peptic ulcer.

Interactions
* *Warfarin*: this increases the risk of haemorrhage if given with fibrinolytic agents.

Route of administration
* IV.

Note
* Patients presenting with acute ischaemic stroke should be thrombolysed if certain criteria are met.
* Fresh frozen plasma with tranexamic acid (an antifibrinolytic agent) may be given if treatment results in excessive bleeding.
* Use of thrombolysis in ST elevation MI is decreasing as primary PCI is the preferred treatment and this is more readably accessible.
* Alteplase and streptokinase can be used in PE. Streptokinase can also be used in DVT, acute arterial thromboembolism, thrombosed arteriovenous shunts and central retinal venous or arterial thrombosis.
* Tenecteplase, alteplase or reteplase are preferred over streptokinase if the patient presents within 6 hours of onset of chest pain with evidence of an anterior MI. They are also used if the patient has had streptokinase in the past because of possible antibodies.

Related drugs
* Alteplase (rt-PA), reteplase, streptokinase, urokinase.

VERAPAMIL

Class: Calcium-channel blocker

Indications
- Hypertension.
- Angina.
- Paroxysmal supraventricular tachycardia.
- Rate control in AF or atrial flutter.

Mechanism of action
- Verapamil inhibits influx of calcium into vascular smooth muscle and myocardium by binding to the L-type calcium channels. This results in:
  1. Relaxation of vascular smooth muscle with subsequent decrease in peripheral resistance and BP.
  2. Decreased myocardial contractility.
  3. Slowed conduction through the AV node and prolonged refractory period (antiarrhythmic properties).
- Angina is relieved by reduction in afterload, heart rate and myocardial contractility, which all reduce myocardial workload.

Adverse effects
- *Common*: constipation, headache, ankle swelling.
- *Rare*: cardiac failure, hypotension, AV-node block.

Contraindications
- Heart failure/cardiogenic shock.
- Hypotension.
- Myocardial conduction defects (e.g. bradycardia, AV-node block, accessory pathway).
- Acute porphyria.

Interactions
- *Amiodarone*: concomitant use of amiodarone and verapamil increases the risk of AV block, bradycardia and myocardial depression.
- *Beta blockers*: if beta blockers are given with, or prior to, verapamil there is an increased risk of AV-node block, which may be complete and result in asystole, heart failure and severe hypotension.
- *Digoxin*: verapamil increases the plasma concentration of digoxin.

Route of administration
- IV (only in paroxysmal tachydysrhythmias), oral.

Note
- Beta blockers are the preferred treatment in unstable angina, as they have been shown to reduce the associated risk of MI. However, if beta blockers are contraindicated or ineffective, verapamil or diltiazem can be used.
- Verapamil and diltiazem should be avoided in heart failure as they can cause marked clinical deterioration due to their negative inotropic effect.

Related drugs
- Diltiazem.

WARFARIN

Class: Oral anticoagulant (vitamin K antagonist)

Indications
- Prevention of thromboembolism (e.g. in AF, prosthetic heart valves).
- Treatment and prevention of DVT and PE.
- Prevention of TIAs and ischaemic stroke in selected patients.

Mechanism of action
- Vitamin K is an essential cofactor for synthesis of clotting factors II, VII, IX and X, and proteins C and S. Warfarin inhibits reduction of vitamin K by inhibiting the enzyme vitamin K epoxide reductase, thereby reducing production of the clotting factors.
- Warfarin takes at least 48–72 hours to achieve its full anticoagulant effect (this reflects the half-life of the clotting factors).

Adverse effects
- *Common*: haemorrhage.
- *Rare*: skin necrosis, liver impairment, alopecia, acute pancreatitis, rash.

Contraindications
- Pregnancy.
- Severe hypertension.
- Active peptic ulcer disease.

Interactions
- *Alcohol, amiodarone, cimetidine, omeprazole, simvastatin*: these increase the anticoagulant effect of warfarin.
- *Aspirin, clopidogrel*: increased risk of haemorrhage.
- *Carbamazepine, rifampicin, spironolactone*: these decrease the anticoagulant effect of warfarin.
- *Combined oral contraceptive (COC) pill*: decreased anticoagulant effect.
- *Note*: warfarin is metabolized by hepatic enzymes that can be induced or inhibited by other drugs, hence a wide range of further interactions exists.

Route of administration
- Oral.

Note
- Therapy should be assessed regularly by measuring INR. The target INR varies with different conditions.
- Warfarin may rarely cause fetal abnormalities if taken during pregnancy (e.g. chondrodysplasia punctata), particularly in the first trimester, and also increases risk of fetal bleeding during delivery hence only used in special circumstances in pregnancy.
- In severe haemorrhage warfarin should be stopped and IV vitamin K with clotting factors II, VII, IX and X should be given. If clotting factors are unavailable, fresh frozen plasma can be used.
- Usually heparin is continued until the therapeutic INR has been achieved with warfarin.
- Over-anticoagulation usually results from a drug interaction with an antibiotic or certain foods.

Related drugs
- Dabigatran, nicoumalone, phenindione.

RESPIRATORY SYSTEM

Management guidelines

ASTHMA
Acute asthma
- Treatment must not be delayed for investigations.
- Therapy is guided by clinical state (i.e. heart rate, respiratory rate, ability to complete sentences, oxygen saturations, BP) and peak expiratory flow rate (PEFR) (but patient may be too ill to perform this).
- Give high-flow oxygen through non-rebreathing face mask.
- Give salbutamol via an oxygen-driven nebulizer.
- Give IV hydrocortisone or oral prednisolone.
- Perform an arterial blood gas if there are life-threatening features: PEFR <33% of best or predicted, oxygen saturation <92%, silent chest, feeble respiratory effort, bradycardia, dysrhythmia, exhaustion, hypotension, confusion, coma.
- Perform a CXR to exclude pneumothorax, infection and other conditions.
- Check response to treatment by monitoring oxygen saturation, PEFR, respiratory rate and arterial blood gas.
- If the patient fails to respond to treatment or is deteriorating:
  - Add ipratropium bromide nebulizer and administer salbutamol nebulizers more frequently (e.g. salbutamol up to every 15 minutes).

The Hands–on Guide to Clinical Pharmacology, 3rd Edition. By S Chatu.
Published 2010 by Blackwell Publishing Ltd.

- Consider administering a single dose of IV magnesium sulphate over 30 minutes.
- If no improvement, discuss with senior clinician and ITU team and consider IV aminophylline (loading dose is contraindicated if taking oral theophylline) or IV salbutamol.
- If, despite this, the patient fails to improve (especially if P_{CO_2} is rising) transfer to ITU to consider mechanical ventilation.
- If the patient is improving, conduct the following until stabilized:
  - Give oxygen and 4-hourly nebulized salbutamol and 6-hourly nebulized ipratropium bromide.
  - Give daily oral prednisolone for at least 5 days.
  - Wean off nebulizers and transfer to inhaled therapy.
  - Prescribe antibiotics if infective exacerbation.
- Before discharging from hospital, consider stepping up the patient's usual treatment (see Chronic asthma), educate about compliance and check inhaler technique.

Chronic asthma

- Educate, avoid known triggers (e.g. pollen, cats, beta blockers), review regularly, check inhaler technique and compliance.
- Bronchodilators can be delivered via inhalers, spacers and nebulizers.
- Start therapy at appropriate step and proceed to the next step if treatment fails to control symptoms:
  - Step 1: Inhaled beta$_2$ agonist, e.g. salbutamol as required but if needed more than twice weekly this suggests poor control so move on to next step.
  - Step 2: Add regular low-dose inhaled corticosteroid (e.g. beclometasone).
  - Step 3: Add regular inhaled long-acting beta agonist (LABA). However, if beneficial but control is still inadequate, continue LABA but also increase inhaled corticosteroid dose. If no response to LABA, stop it and increase inhaled corticosteroid dose.
  - Step 4: Consider trials of the following and refer for specialist care:
    1. Oral leukotriene antagonist (e.g. montelukast).
    2. Maximum dose inhaled corticosteroids.
    3. Oral theophylline.
  - Step 5: Add regular oral corticosteroid (prednisolone), maximize other treatments and refer for specialist care.
- Review treatment every 3–6 months and titrate steroid dose to the lowest possible for asthma control.

CHRONIC OBSTRUCTIVE PULMONARY DISEASE (COPD)

- Advise to stop smoking and offer help at every opportunity.
- Spirometry is essential to make an accurate diagnosis, assess disease severity and to monitor progression.

- Use short-acting bronchodilators (beta$_2$ agonist and/or anticholinergic) as required to help symptoms and increase exercise tolerance.
- If still symptomatic, switch to a combination of long-acting bronchodilators (beta$_2$ agonist and anticholinergic).
- Use of inhaled corticosteroids:
  - Inhaled corticosteroids should be used in patients with forced expiratory volume in 1 second (FEV$_1$) ≤50% predicted and a history of two or more exacerbations requiring antibiotics or oral corticosteroids in the past year.
- Consider oral theophylline (bronchodilator) if still symptomatic.
- Use mucolytics if chronic productive cough.
- Acute hospital admission:
  - Regular nebulized bronchodilators (i.e. ipratropium, salbutamol).
  - Measure ABGs:
    ○ If hypoxia is present, administer up to 28% oxygen with repeated blood gases.
    ○ If hypercapnia is present with respiratory acidosis, decide if ventilatory support (i.e. non-invasive ventilation, intubation) is appropriate and decide on ceiling of treatment.
  - CXR to assess for pneumothorax, infection and other conditions.
  - For infective acute exacerbations, add appropriate antibiotics and give oral prednisolone for 7–14 days.
  - Chest physiotherapy to prevent accumulation of secretions.
- COPD in the community:
  - Diuretics for any associated cor pulmonale (right-sided heart failure secondary to chronic lung disease).
  - Long-term oxygen therapy in non-smokers if P_{O_2} <7.3 kPa on more than one occasion when clinically stable or P_{O_2} = 7.3–8.0 with pulmonary hypertension or secondary polycythaemia.
  - Influenza and pneumococcal vaccine should be offered.
  - Pulmonary rehabilitation offered (e.g. disease education, physical training).
  - Consider surgery for selected patients, i.e. lung transplant, volume reduction surgery and bullectomy.
  - Advisable to have course of steroids and antibiotics at home for acute exacerbations to avoid hospital admission.

SMOKING CESSATION
- Smoking cessation reduces ill health and prolongs life.
- Advise stopping at every opportunity.
- Once target stop date agreed, prescribe nicotine replacement therapy or bupropion for 2–4 weeks with access to support groups.
- Varenicline (selective nicotine receptor partial agonist) can be used to help stop smoking for 1–2 weeks before target stop date.

Drugs

BECLOMETASONE

Class: Corticosteroid

Indications
- Prophylaxis of asthma.
- Symptomatic relief in COPD.
- Inflammatory skin disorders (e.g. eczema, psoriasis).
- Prophylaxis and treatment of allergic or vasomotor rhinitis.
- Mild–moderate ulcerative colitis.

Mechanism of action
- Corticosteroids act on cell receptors to modify gene function causing a multitude of effects that inhibit inflammation and immune processes. They suppress T-lymphocytes and expression of cytokines. They inhibit neutrophil action and have other unknown mechanisms.
- In asthma, corticosteroids act by reducing airway inflammation, which leads to decreased oedema and decreased mucus secretion.

Adverse effects
- *Common*: cough and oral candidiasis (with inhaled route); nasal irritation (with nasal spray); thinning of the skin (with topical treatment).
- *Rare*: hoarse voice (with inhaled route); nose bleeds, disturbance of smell (with long-term nasal spray); acne and depigmentation at the site of application (with topical treatment); glaucoma, cataract.

Contraindications
- Skin ointment is contraindicated in acne vulgaris, rosacea and skin infections.
- Nasal spray is contraindicated in untreated nasal infections and during the recovery phase post nasal surgery.

Interactions
- Nil significant.

Route of administration
- Inhalation (asthma), topical (skin conditions), nasal spray (rhinitis), tablet (ulcerative colitis, oral aphthous ulcers).

Note
- Using a spacer with the inhaler can prevent oral candidiasis and hoarseness. Additionally, the mouth can be rinsed out with water after using the inhaler.
- Current and ex-smokers usually need higher doses of inhaled steroids due to reduced effectiveness.
- Oral budesonide can be used in the treatment of inflammatory bowel disease and microscopic colitis.

Related drugs
- Budesonide, ciclesonide, fluticasone, mometasone.

IPRATROPIUM BROMIDE

Class: Muscarinic antagonist

Indications
- COPD.
- Asthma (acute and chronic).
- Rhinorrhoea.

Mechanism of action
- It acts locally by blocking muscarinic receptors in bronchial smooth muscle leading to bronchodilatation and a reduction in bronchial mucus secretion.
- When applied as a nasal spray, ipratropium inhibits secretions from seromucus glands lining the nasal mucosa.

Adverse effects
- *Common*: headache, dizziness, cough, dry mouth.
- *Rare*: urinary retention, rash, glaucoma (with nebulized route).

Contraindications
- None.
- Caution:
  - Glaucoma.
  - Pregnancy and breastfeeding.
  - Bladder outflow obstruction.
  - BPH.

Interactions
- No significant interactions.

Route of administration
- Inhalation (aerosol, powder, nebulized solution), nasal spray.

Note
- Ipratropium is a polar molecule that is poorly absorbed and thus has very few systemic effects. However, if administered via a nebulizer, it can cause glaucoma through a direct topical effect on the eyes, hence protection goggles are advised.
- Ipratropium is thought to be more effective in relieving bronchoconstriction in COPD than in asthma.
- Risk of urinary retention is increased if there is pre-existing urinary outflow obstruction.
- Tiotropium is a long-acting muscarinic antagonist used as once-daily maintenance treatment in COPD.

Related drugs
- Oxitropium, tiotropium.

MONTELUKAST

Class: Leukotriene-receptor antagonist

Indications
* Treatment of chronic asthma.
* Allergic rhinitis.

Mechanism of action
* Montelukast is a selective, competitive antagonist at cysteinyl leukotriene receptors. Leukotrienes are released as part of an inflammatory and allergic reaction, e.g. asthma, and are potent bronchoconstrictors. This drug blocks action of leukotrienes on receptors in the lungs and airways, thus reducing bronchoconstriction and mucus secretion.

Adverse effects
* *Common*: headache, dizziness, rash, dyspepsia, abdominal pain.
* *Rare*: anaphylaxis, sleep disorders, palpitations.

Contraindications
* None.
* Caution:
  * Churg–Strauss syndrome (may be exacerbated by montelukast).
  * Pregnancy.
  * Breastfeeding.

Interactions
* *Phenobarbital, primidone*: reduce the plasma concentration of montelukast.

Route of administration
* Oral.

Note
* Montelukast is no more effective than inhaled corticosteroids in the management of chronic asthma. However, when used together, these two drugs have an additive effect.
* Montelukast should not be used in the management of acute asthma.
* The use of montelukast has been associated with Churg–Strauss syndrome.
* Montelukast is extensively metabolized by hepatic cytochrome P450 enzymes.
* Montelukast can be used in the treatment of eosinophilic oesophagitis.

Related drugs
* Zafirlukast.

NICOTINE

Class: Nicotine

Indications
* Smoking cessation.

Mechanism of action
* Nicotine replacement therapy (NRT) stops or reduces symptoms of nicotine withdrawal, enabling one to stop smoking without withdrawal symptoms. With NRT one is not exposed to harmful chemicals from cigarettes.

Adverse effects
* *Common*: nausea, dyspepsia, dry mouth, headache, dizziness, rash.
* *Rare*: palpitations, sleep disturbance.

Contraindications
* Caution:
  * Recent MI, stroke and arrhythmias.
  * Pregnancy and breastfeeding; however, the risk of harm from cigarettes is more than from NRT.

Interactions
* *Theophylline*: NRT will increase levels of this drug hence dose should be reduced.

Route of administration
* Lozenges, sublingual tablet, patches, gum, inhaled, nasal spray.

Note
* To maintain abstinence from cigarettes, should have support or counselling while on NRT.
* Patient preference determines route of administration.
* If withdrawal symptoms are severe then patches can be combined with gum or nasal spray
* Dose of NRT is usually reduced in the latter part of the course and then stopped

OXYGEN

Class: Therapeutic gas

Indications
*   High concentrations (mask with reservoir bag can deliver up to 85% oxygen, endotracheal tube can deliver 100% oxygen) for acute hypoxic events (e.g. MI, acute asthma, PE).
*   Low concentrations (up to 28% oxygen) in patients with respiratory disease with carbon dioxide retention (e.g. COPD).

Mechanism of action
*   Oxygen specifically binds to haemoglobin and also dissolves in plasma. It is then transported to tissues, where it promotes aerobic respiration.
*   In hypoxaemic patients, oxygen decreases the work of breathing needed to maintain arterial oxygen saturation.

Adverse effects
*   *Rare*: retinopathy in neonates (with high concentrations), respiratory arrest in COPD due to loss of hypoxic drive, pulmonary oedema.

Contraindications
*   None.

Interactions
*   None known.

Route of administration
*   Nasal cannulae, face mask, tent, hood, endotracheal tube.

Note
*   A humidifier should be used when oxygen is administered in high concentrations, as it can cause retrosternal discomfort and dry cough. High-flow oxygen, i.e. 85%, becomes uncomfortable after approximately 12 hours of continuous administration, while 50% oxygen is usually safe for any period of time.
*   Different face masks deliver different concentrations of oxygen: Venturi mask delivers 24–60%; Hudson mask up to 50%; Hudson mask with reservoir bag up to 85%; nasal cannulae up to 35%. Anaesthetic circuit via endotracheal tube can deliver up to 100% oxygen. Endotracheal tube is the only definite means of delivering known concentrations of oxygen.
*   Oxygen should only be prescribed for home use after a thorough medical evaluation. Patients using home oxygen should be advised of fire risks.
*   Long-term home oxygen may prolong survival in patients with severe COPD (at least 15 hours of oxygen should be used per day).
*   Can be prescribed at home for terminally ill patients and in those with chronic respiratory, cardiac or neurological conditions if there is disabling dyspnoea.

SALBUTAMOL

Class: Beta$_2$ agonist

Indications
- Asthma.
- COPD with reversible component.
- Premature labour.

Mechanism of action
- Salbutamol stimulates beta$_2$ adrenoceptors in the airways, thus generating intracellular cyclic adenosine monophosphate (cAMP). This decreases intracellular calcium and produces bronchodilatation (as calcium is required for bronchial smooth muscle contraction).
- Increased cAMP also prevents degranulation of mast cells.
- When used in premature labour, salbutamol acts by inhibiting uterine smooth muscle contraction.

Adverse effects
- *Common*: tremor, tachycardia.
- *Rare*: headache, palpitations, hypokalaemia, muscle cramps, insomnia (these adverse effects are dose dependent and therefore more common with high doses).

Contraindications
- None.

Interactions
- *Corticosteroids*: high doses of corticosteroids given with high doses of salbutamol increase the risk of hypokalaemia.
- *Diuretics*: high doses of salbutamol increase the risk of hypokalaemia if given with loop or thiazide diuretics.
- *Theophylline*: high doses of salbutamol increase the risk of hypokalaemia if given with theophylline.

Route of administration
- Asthma: inhalation (aerosol, powder, nebulized solution), IM, IV, oral.
- COPD: inhalation.
- Premature labour: IM or IV.

Note
- Plasma potassium needs to be monitored if salbutamol is given in severe asthma. This is due to the increased risk of hypokalaemia caused by high doses of salbutamol and concomitant treatment with diuretics and theophylline.
- Metered-dose inhalers are only useful in patients over 8 years of age. If younger, a spacer should be used to administer inhaled salbutamol; this is also useful in adults with poor inhaler technique.
- LABAs are available in combination with inhaled corticosteroids for treatment of chronic asthma and COPD.

Related drugs
- Short-acting beta$_2$ antagonists: bambuterol, fenoterol, reproterol, terbutaline, tulobuterol.
- LABAs: formoterol, salmeterol.

SODIUM CROMOGLICATE

Class: Mast cell stabilizer

Indications
* Prophylaxis of asthma.
* Allergic rhinitis.
* Allergic conjunctivitis.
* Food allergy.

Mechanism of action
* Exact mechanism is not fully understood.
* Sodium cromoglicate may reduce calcium influx into mast cells, thus rendering them more stable, i.e. less likely to release inflammatory mediators. This occurs in the bronchial tree, the nose and the eyes.

Adverse effects
* *Common*: cough, throat irritation, stinging of the eyes (with eye drops).
* *Rare*: nausea, vomiting, joint pain, rash (all with oral administration); transient bronchospasm (with inhaled route).

Contraindications
* None.

Interactions
* None known.

Route of administration
* Asthma: inhalation (aerosol, powder or nebulized solution).
* Food allergy: oral.
* Allergic rhinitis: nasal spray.
* Allergic conjunctivitis: eye drops.

Note
* Sodium cromoglicate is not used in the acute exacerbation of asthma.
* Roughly one-third of patients taking sodium cromoglicate, especially children, benefit from it.
* Sodium cromoglicate is generally less effective than inhaled corticosteroids in the prophylaxis of asthma in adults and is therefore not commonly used.
* Sodium cromoglicate is useful in the prevention of exercise-induced asthma.
* If transient bronchospasm is a problematic adverse effect, a $beta_2$ agonist can be inhaled a few minutes before sodium cromoglicate.
* Throat irritation can be avoided by rinsing the mouth with water after inhalation.

Related drugs
* Nedocromil sodium.

THEOPHYLLINE

Class: Methylxanthine

Indications
- Asthma.

Mechanism of action
- Bronchodilatation is thought to be achieved by a variety of mechanisms, including inhibition of the enzyme phosphodiesterase, which degrades cAMP. The raised cAMP levels subsequently decrease intracellular calcium, resulting in bronchodilatation.
- Theophylline also blocks adenosine receptors, which results in smooth muscle relaxation in the bronchi.
- Theophylline increases the force of contraction of the diaphragm, possibly by enhancing calcium uptake.
- Theophylline is further believed to inhibit inflammatory cells, such as mast cells.

Adverse effects
- *Common*: nausea, vomiting, headache, palpitations, tachycardia.
- *Rare*: hypokalaemia, diarrhoea, central nervous system (CNS) stimulation (insomnia, irritability, fine tremor), convulsions, dysrhythmias.

Contraindications
- None.
- Caution:
  - Cardiac disease (risk of dysrhythmias).
  - Hypertension.
  - Epilepsy.

Interactions
- *Ciprofloxacin, erythromycin*: these increase the plasma concentration of theophylline.
- *Diltiazem, verapamil*: these increase the plasma concentration of theophylline.
- *Note*: theophylline is metabolized by hepatic enzymes that can be induced or inhibited by other drugs; hence a wide range of further interactions exists.

Route of administration
- IV (as aminophylline, in acute severe asthma), oral.

Note
- Therapeutic drug monitoring is recommended.
- Oral sustained-release tablets are available which are effective for up to 12 hours (less adverse effects).
- Theophylline can be given in combination with ethylenediamine as aminophylline. This is more readily absorbed and has fewer GI adverse effects.
- Theophylline and aminophylline should not be given together due to the risk of serious adverse effects (e.g. convulsions or dysrhythmias).
- Aminophylline or theophylline are used in COPD patients who have a component of reversible airways obstruction.

Related drugs
- Aminophylline.

GASTROINTESTINAL SYSTEM

The Hands–on Guide to Clinical Pharmacology, 3rd Edition. By S Chatu.
Published 2010 by Blackwell Publishing Ltd.

Management guidelines

CONSTIPATION
*   Exclude underlying pathology with history, examination and appropriate investigations.
*   Treat any underlying cause, e.g. colonic obstruction from tumour, diverticular stricture, drug induced, hypothyroidism and hypercalcaemia.
*   If no organic pathology is found, the usual cause is idiopathic constipation or due to irritable bowel syndrome.
*   Recommend high-fibre diet with adequate fluid intake.
*   If the above fails, consider any of the following laxatives with regular review:
    *   *Bulking agents* (ispaghula husk, methylcellulose, sterculia) increase faecal mass, which stimulates peristalsis.
    *   *Osmotic laxatives* (lactulose, macrogols, magnesium salts, phosphate enema) increase amount of water in large bowel.
    *   *Stimulant laxatives* (bisacodyl, dantron, docusate sodium, glycerol suppositories, senna, sodium picosulphate) increase intestinal motility.
    *   *Stool softener* – arachis oil enema is rarely used in faecal impaction.
*   In some situations, consider behavioural treatments such as biofeedback therapy, psychological support, pelvic floor exercises, dietary and lifestyle advice.
*   In extreme cases, a colectomy with an ileostomy or ileo-rectal anastomosis may be considered.

DIARRHOEA
*   Remember that most cases of diarrhoea are self-limiting and often caused by viruses (e.g. rotavirus).
*   Antibiotics are not usually required for simple gastroenteritis.
*   Aim of treatment is to replace fluid and electrolyte losses by oral rehydration therapy (IV in nausea and vomiting).
*   The following can be given for symptomatic relief in uncomplicated acute diarrhoea in adults (but rule out infectious diarrhoea with stool samples first):
    *   Loperamide.
    *   Codeine phosphate.
    *   Diphenoxylate.
    *   *Note*: antimotility agents should not be used in the management of acute diarrhoea in children.
*   Common bacterial causes of diarrhoea are *Campylobacter* spp., *Shigella* spp. and *Giardia* spp. See p. 162 for treatment.
*   If clinically indicated, diarrhoea persisting for more than 2 weeks with negative stool cultures should be investigated further with lower GI tract endoscopy, blood tests (i.e. thyroid profile, coeliac serology) and radiological investigations.

INFLAMMATORY BOWEL DISEASE

Crohn's disease

- This condition can affect any part of the GI tract from the mouth to the anus. Therefore, therapy is tailored to the individual.
- Administer a 5-ASA preparation (e.g. mesalazine, sulfasalazine) to help maintain remission.
- Treat infective complications such as abscesses with antibiotics, e.g. metronidazole, ciprofloxacin.
- Administer corticosteroids (e.g. budesonide or prednisolone) orally, rectally or IV depending on disease extent and severity until symptoms resolve. Not to be used for maintenance due to adverse effects.
- Consider elemental diet or parenteral nutrition to allow bowel rest and help induce remission in a flare up.
- If no improvement with above therapy, consider starting immunosuppressants (azathioprine, mercaptopurine, methotrexate).
- In some cases, biological therapies (adalimumab, infliximab, natalizumab) are effective in maintaining remission.
- Hospitalized patients with active disease should receive prophylactic heparin because of increased risk of venous and arterial thrombosis due to increased clotting factors and often an elevated platelet count.
- Small bowel involvement may lead to iron, folate and vitamin B_{12} deficiencies; those should be replaced.
- Surgery may be required for bowel obstruction, perforation, perianal disease, haemorrhage or fistula formation.

Ulcerative colitis
Maintenance of remission

- Give a 5-ASA preparation as maintenance therapy (e.g. mesalazine, sulfasalazine) orally or rectally, depending on disease extent and severity.
- Rectal suppositories are ideal if disease is confined to the recto-sigmoid junction; rectal enemas are effective for left-sided disease up to the splenic flexure.
- Oral and topical treatment with 5-ASA drugs are combined for more extensive disease.
- In some individuals remission is maintained with immunosuppressants (i.e. azathioprine, mercaptopurine, methotrexate), especially in steroid-dependent or resistant cases.
- In resistant cases, biologics can be used, e.g. infliximab to induce and maintain remission.

Acute flare

- Add systemic corticosteroids orally, rectally or IV in acute ulcerative colitis not responding to maximum dose of 5-ASA and stop when in remission.
- If still no improvement, patient should be admitted for IV corticosteroids.
- If there is no improvement after 5 days of corticosteroid therapy, providing infective causes of diarrhoea have been excluded, consider IV ciclosporin or biologic therapy, e.g. infliximab.

- If still no improvement, consider surgery.
- Hospitalized patients with active disease should receive prophylactic heparin because of increased risk of venous and arterial thrombosis, due to increased clotting factors and often an elevated platelet count.

IRRITABLE BOWEL SYNDROME

- General dietary advice, physical activity and symptom-targeted medication are the principles of treatment.
- Referral to a dietitian for advice about elimination diets can relieve symptoms.
- Pharmacological treatments with antispasmodics taken as required for abdominal pain, laxatives for constipation and loperamide for diarrhoea, with dose adjustment to maintain soft well-formed stool may be adequate.
- Consider amitriptyline for its analgesic effect if laxatives, loperamide or antispasmodics are ineffective; SSRIs may be used where amitriptyline is intolerable or ineffective.
- Consider psychological intervention if dietary and pharmacological intervention ineffective, i.e. cognitive behavioural therapy (CBT), hypnotherapy and psychological therapy.

NAUSEA AND VOMITING

- While an underlying cause is being established, antiemetics provide symptomatic relief and there are many types available.
- Causes of nausea and vomiting include:
  - GI pathology, drug/toxin induced, motion sickness, pregnancy, intracranial pathology, psychogenic, pain, systemic illness, metabolic disturbance, vestibular disease.
- The following drugs act on the brainstem to help resolve symptoms:
  1. Antihistamines (cinnarizine, cyclizine, promethazine).
  2. Anticholinergic (hyoscine).
  3. Dopamine antagonists (chlorpromazine, domperidone, metoclopramide, prochlorperazine, trifluoperazine).
  4. Serotonin antagonists (dolasetron, granisetron, ondansetron, palonosetron, tropisetron).
  5. Cannabinoid (nabilone).
  6. Neurokinin-receptor antagonists (aprepitant, fosaprepitant).
  7. Dexamethasone.
  8. Betahistine.

GASTRO-OESOPHAGEAL REFLUX DISEASE

- Avoid or cut down on foods that trigger symptoms.
- Leave at least 3–4 hours between the evening meal and bedtime.
- Weight reduction, avoiding excess alcohol, caffeine and stopping smoking may help.
- For nocturnal symptoms elevate the end of the bed.
- If the above fail, use an antacid/alginate as required.
- For daily symptoms, advise regular H_2 antagonist (e.g. ranitidine).
- If no response, start a PPI (e.g. omeprazole).

- If still symptomatic on maximum dose PPI, can add a H_2 antagonist at night in combination with an antacid/alginate after meals.
- Consider adding drugs that improve gut motility and oesophageal clearance, e.g. domperidone or metoclopramide.
- If still symptomatic, consider surgical intervention, e.g. nissen fundoplication.

PEPTIC ULCER DISEASE

- Most gastric ulcers (70–75%) and nearly all duodenal ulcers (90%) are caused by *Helicobacter pylori* infection. The rest are due to NSAIDs.
- Stop NSAIDs (if appropriate).
- Reduce exacerbating factors (e.g. smoking, obesity, alcohol, spicy foods). However, these measures have been less important since the discovery of *H. pylori*.
- Administer triple therapy for *H. pylori* infection (if appropriate).
- A PPI (e.g. omeprazole) given for 4 weeks should heal 90% of duodenal ulcers; it should also heal 80–90% of gastric ulcers if given for 8 weeks.
- H_2 antagonists (e.g. ranitidine) are less effective than PPIs and are not routinely used for the treatment of peptic ulcers.
- Other ulcer-healing agents include bismuth and sucralfate.
- In resistant cases, consider surgery (e.g. vagotomy $+/-$ pyloroplasty for a duodenal ulcer; partial gastrectomy for a gastric ulcer)
- If a gastric ulcer is found, important to repeat the endoscopy at 6 weeks, to make sure it is healing and not malignant.

Helicobacter pylori infection eradication

- Important to eradicate in the presence of a peptic ulcer to prevent recurrence.
- Confirm the presence of *H. pylori* prior to starting eradication treatment (i.e. serology, ^{13}C-urea breath test, stool test, histology from gastric biopsies, CLOtest®).
- Triple therapy (PPI + clarithromycin + amoxicillin *or* PPI + clarithromycin + metronidazole) for 1 week eradicates *H. pylori* in 80–85% of cases.
- If patient has used clarithromycin or metronidazole in the past year for an infection, use an alternative as resistance is common.
- Treatment failure is usually due to poor compliance or resistance to antibiotics.
- If symptomatic after eradication, arrange a urea breath test or stool test and treat with quadruple therapy if positive.
- Quadruple therapy involves a PPI + bismuth + tetracycline + *either* metronidazole *or* tinidazole for 1 week.

HEPATITIS B

- Treatment in chronic hepatitis B infection should be considered if there is evidence of active viral replication and either persistent elevation in serum aminotransferases (alanine transaminase [ALT], aspartate transaminase [AST]) or histological active disease.

- Treatment is with peginterferon alfa or interferon alfa as initial therapy. If this is poorly tolerated or there is no response, a nucleoside/nucleotide analogue can be used.
- A nucleoside/nucleotide can be used as monotherapy in all stages of liver disease.

HEPATITIS C

- Treatment is with peginterferon alfa (interferon alfa is an alternative but not commonly used) given weekly by subcutaneous injection in combination with oral ribavirin.
- Peginterferon should be used alone if ribavirin is contraindicated or not tolerated.
- Duration of treatment depends on the genotype; currently 24 weeks for genotype 2 and 3 and 48 weeks for genotypes 1, 4, 5 and 6.
- Protease inhibitors and polymerase inhibitors, known as specifically targeted antiviral therapy for hepatitis C (STAT-C), are currently in clinical trials and appear promising.

Drugs

ANTACIDS/ALGINATES

(Aluminium salts, magnesium salts)

Indications
- Symptomatic relief of:
  - Ulcer dyspepsia.
  - Gastro-oesophageal reflux disease.

Mechanism of action
- Antacids are weak alkalis that neutralize the acid in the stomach.
- Some antacids are combined with alginates to further suppress acid reflux. Alginates protect the oesophagus by forming a 'raft', which decreases acid regurgitation.
- The antacid/alginate combination also prevents non-acid reflux by protecting the oesophageal mucosa from bile and pepsin, which is thought to be beneficial.

Adverse effects
- *Common*: constipation (aluminium salts), diarrhoea (magnesium salts).

Contraindications
- Hypophosphataemia (aluminium and magnesium salts).
- Caution:
  - Renal impairment (magnesium salts).

Interactions
- *ACE inhibitors, antibacterials, digoxin, iron*: antacids decrease the absorption of these drugs.
- *Lithium*: sodium bicarbonate increases the excretion of lithium.

Route of administration
- Oral.

Note
- Usually taken when symptomatic or after meals and before bedtime to prevent expected symptoms.
- Most antacids are not absorbed from the GI tract and therefore rarely cause systemic adverse effects.
- Simeticone (antifoaming agent) can be added to antacids to reduce flatulence.
- Preparations containing more than one antacid do not have a superior effect in comparison to simple preparations.

ANTISPASMODICS

(Dicyclomine hydrochloride – Bentyl®, hyoscine butylbromide – Buscopan®)

Class: Antimuscarinics

Indications
* Symptomatic relief of symptoms in irritable bowel syndrome.

Mechanism of action
* Relax intestinal smooth muscle and reduce intestinal motility by acting on the parasympathetic nervous system in the gut.
* May help in relieving cramping abdominal pain due to gut spasm after meals or occurring unexpectedly.

Adverse effects
* *Common*: dry mouth, constipation.
* *Rare*: urinary urgency and retention, closed-angle glaucoma, blurred vision.

Contraindications
* Myasthenia gravis.
* Paralytic ileus.
* Closed-angle glaucoma.
* Prostatic enlargement.

Interactions
* Nil significant.

Route of administration
* Oral.
* Buscopan®: oral, IM, IV.

Note
* The response to antispasmodics varies in individuals; however, they are well tolerated.
* Usually taken before meals to prevent anticipated abdominal pain or when required.
* Buscopan is used to facilitate radiological and endoscopic procedures where spasm may be a problem.
* Alverine citrate (Spasmonal®), Mebeverine® and peppermint oil capsules are direct relaxants of smooth muscle which can also be used in irritable bowel syndrome.

Related drugs
* Alverine citrate (Spasmonal®), Mebeverine®, peppermint oil capsules.

5-AMINOSALICYLATES (5- ASAs)

(Balsalazide, mesalazine, olsalazine, sulfasalazine)

Class: Aminosalicylate

Indications
- Treatment and maintenance of ulcerative colitis.
- Treatment of Crohn's disease.
- Rheumatoid arthritis (only sulfasalazine).

Mechanism of action
- Sulfasalazine is split into 5-ASA and sulfapyridine (a sulfonamide) by colonic flora. The function of sulfapyridine is to carry 5-ASA to the gut. 5-ASA has an anti-inflammatory action in the large bowel. The other 5-ASA drugs are released in the small or large bowel by different mechanisms.
- In rheumatoid arthritis, it is the sulfapyridine component that acts as a disease-modifying antirheumatic drug.

Adverse effects
- *Common*: nausea, abdominal discomfort, diarrhoea, headache, rash.
- *Rare*: blood dyscrasias (i.e. aplastic anaemia, leucopenia, thrombocytopenia), acute pancreatitis, hepatitis, renal impairment (interstitial nephritis, nephrotic syndrome), lupus erythematosus-like syndrome, alopecia, cardiac effects (myocarditis, pericarditis), allergic lung reactions, peripheral neuropathy.

Contraindications
- Salicylate hypersensitivity.
- Renal impairment.
- Children under the age of 2 years.

Interactions
- No significant interactions.

Route of administration
- Oral, rectal enema or suppository.

Note
- Sulfasalazine causes reversible oligospermia and balsalazide is not recommended in pregnancy, hence an alternative should be used if patient is planning to start a family.
- 5-ASAs can rarely exacerbate colitis.
- As 5-ASAs can cause blood dyscrasias, patients should be advised to report any unexplained bleeding, bruising or sore throat. If these symptoms occur, a FBC should be performed immediately.
- Owing to risk of renal, liver and blood disorders, monitoring of FBC, LFTs and renal function with urinalysis to exclude nephrotic syndrome is recommended 6–12 monthly.
- 5-ASA drugs are prescribed by brand name as they differ in terms of mechanism of action, dose and costs. Common preparations used are Asacol®, Colazide®, Mezavant®, Pentasa® and Salofalk®.

ADEFOVIR

Class: Nucleotide analogue

Indications
* Treatment of chronic hepatitis B infection.

Mechanism of action
* Adefovir blocks the enzyme reverse transcriptase required for hepatitis B virus replication in the body.

Adverse effects
* *Common*: nausea.
* *Rare*: asthenia, headache, renal failure, hypophosphataemia.

Contraindications
* Breastfeeding.

Interactions
* Nil.

Route of administration
* Oral.

Note
* During therapy, patients may develop lactic acidosis, hepatitis and renal failure so clinical and biochemical monitoring is required.
* Can develop a severe hepatitis following cessation of therapy with nucleoside/nucleotide drugs.
* Peginterferon alfa is recommended for initial treatment in chronic hepatitis B infection. A nucleoside/nucleotide analogue can be used if there is no response to peginterferon or it is poorly tolerated of contraindicated.
* The nucleotide/nucleoside analogues can be used as monotherapy in all stages of liver disease.
* Lamivudine is often used first line when peginterferon is inappropriate; however, long-term use is associated with viral resistance requiring either addition or switching to another nucleoside/nucleotide drug.

Related drugs
* Nucleoside analogue: entecavir, lamivudine, telbivudine.
* Nucleotide analogue: tenofovir.

CICLOSPORIN

Class: Immunosuppressive agent

Indications
- Inflammatory bowel disease.
- Prevention of transplant rejection.
- Prophylaxis and treatment of graft-versus-host disease.
- Nephrotic syndrome.
- Severe eczema and psoriasis (when conventional therapy has failed).

Mechanism of action
- Ciclosporin is an immunosuppressive agent directed mainly against T lymphocytes. It prevents their activation and reduces the release of cytokines, in particular interleukin-2. This action suppresses cell-mediated immunity and, to a lesser extent, antibody-mediated immunity.

Adverse effects
- *Common*: nephrotoxicity, hypertension.
- *Rare*: hirsutism, gum hypertrophy, seizures, muscle weakness, hepatic impairment.

Contraindications
- Renal disease.
- Liver disease.
- Uncontrolled hypertension.
- Malignancy.

Interactions
- *Aminoglycosides, erythromycin, trimethoprim*: these drugs increase plasma ciclosporin levels, thus increasing the risk of nephrotoxicity.
- *Carbamazepine, phenytoin, rifampicin*: these drugs reduce the plasma concentration of ciclosporin.
- *Diltiazem, verapamil*: these drugs increase the plasma concentration of ciclosporin, thus increasing the risk of nephrotoxicity.
- *NSAIDs*: concomitant use of NSAIDs and ciclosporin increases the risk of nephrotoxicity.

Route of administration
- Oral, IV.

Note
- Unlike other immunosuppressive agents, ciclosporin does not cause bone marrow suppression.
- Therapeutic drug monitoring is required.
- Some evidence suggests that patients taking ciclosporin are at an increased risk of secondary lymphomas caused by Epstein–Barr virus (EBV) infection. This is believed to be due to impaired immunity.
- Before starting IV ciclosporin in acute ulcerative colitis refractory to corticosteroids, it is important to check magnesium and cholesterol as low levels increase risk of seizures.
- Grapefruit juice should be avoided as it increases ciclosporin levels and thus toxicity.

COLESTYRAMINE

Class: Bile acid sequestrant

Indications
* Hypercholesterolaemia.
* To prevent diarrhoea in bile acid malabsorption (terminal ileal Crohn's or resection, post cholecystectomy, primary bile salt malabsorption).
* Prevent pruritus secondary to bile duct obstruction, e.g. primary biliary cirrhosis, primary sclerosing cholangitis.

Mechanism of action
* Removes bile acids from the body by forming insoluble complexes with bile acids in the GI tract which are then excreted in stool. This prevents reabsorption of bile acids.
* The reduction in bile acid levels promotes cholesterol conversion to bile acids by the liver thereby leading to increased LDL-cholesterol uptake from the plasma to compensate, leading to a reduction in plasma LDL-cholesterol levels.
* Binding of bile acids in the GI tract prevents their irritant effect on the colon, preventing diarrhoea.

Adverse effects
* *Common*: constipation, abdominal discomfort, flatulence.
* *Rare*: diarrhoea, bleeding due to vitamin K deficiency.

Contraindications
* Intestinal obstruction.

Interactions
* Prevents absorption of many drugs; take other drugs either 1 hour before or 4–6 hours after colestyramine.

Route of administration
* Oral.

Note
* If colestyramine is not tolerated because of its GI side-effects use alternative bile acid sequestrants that are better tolerated, such as colestipol or colesevelam.
* Colestyramine is a powder that is mixed with fruit juice, milk or water prior to ingestion.

Related drugs
* Colesevelam, colestipol.

CYCLIZINE

Class: Histamine$_1$ (H$_1$)-receptor antagonist

Indications
* Nausea and vomiting.
* Labyrinthine disturbances causing nausea and vomiting.
* Motion sickness.

Mechanism of action
* Cyclizine acts as a competitive antagonist at H$_1$ receptors in the vomiting centre of the brain.
* It also has weak antimuscarinic effects and is mildly sedating.

Adverse effects
* *Common*: headache.
* *Rare*: insomnia, palpitations, antimuscarinic effects (e.g. urinary retention, dry mouth), drowsiness.

Contraindications
* Acute porphyria
* Caution:
    * Urinary retention and BPH (antihistamines have antimuscarinic effects).

Interactions
* *Alcohol*: this enhances the sedative effect of cyclizine.
* *Antimuscarinics*: these enhance the antimuscarinic effects of cyclizine.

Route of administration
* Oral, IM, IV.

Note
* Antiemetics should only be administered when the cause of nausea is known, as they may otherwise delay diagnosis.
* A combination of two antiemetics with different sites of action may be effective in nausea and vomiting that is not alleviated by a single agent.
* Unlike metoclopramide, cyclizine is effective in the treatment of motion sickness.
* Cyclizine is a safe antiemetic in pregnancy.

Related drugs
* Cinnarizine, promethazine.

FERROUS SULPHATE

Class: Iron salt

Indications
* Iron-deficiency anaemia.

Mechanism of action
* Ferrous sulphate replenishes iron stores.

Adverse effects
* *Common*: nausea, epigastric pain, constipation or diarrhoea, darkening of faeces (often confused with melaena).

Contraindications
* None.
* Caution:
  * Pregnancy.

Interactions
* *Magnesium salts*: reduce the absorption of iron.
* *Quinolone antibiotics*: iron reduces absorption of these drugs.
* *Tetracycline*: reduces the absorption of iron.

Route of administration
* Oral.

Note
* The cause of iron-deficiency anaemia should be sought prior to administration of ferrous sulphate. Possible causes are malignancy of the GI tract, coeliac disease, dietary and pregnancy.
* Iron deficiency causes a hypochromic microcytic anaemia with low serum ferritin levels and increased total iron-binding capacity (TIBC).
* Haemoglobin (Hb) concentration increases by roughly 2 g/100 ml with every 3–4 weeks of treatment.
* In order to replenish iron stores, treatment with oral ferrous sulphate is continued for 3–6 months after Hb levels have reached the normal range.
* Patients unable to tolerate oral iron (e.g. because of severe adverse effects) should be given IV iron.
* Absorption of ferrous sulphate can be improved by combining it with vitamin C.
* Potentially fatal iron poisoning, which can cause nausea, vomiting, bloody diarrhoea, haematemesis, abdominal pain, hypotension and coma, is commonest in children.

Related drugs
* Ferrous fumarate, ferrous gluconate.

FOLIC ACID

Class: Vitamin supplement

Indications
*   Prevention of neural tube defects in pregnancy.
*   Folate-deficient megaloblastic anaemia.
*   Chronic haemolytic states.
*   Prevention of folate deficiency in patients taking anticonvulsants (carbamazepine, phenytoin) and methotrexate.

Mechanism of action
*   Folic acid has a role in cell metabolism due to its ability to transfer single carbon-atom-containing groups. This is important in the synthesis of purines and pyrimidines and therefore in the synthesis of DNA.

Adverse effects
*   None.

Contraindications
*   Folic acid alone should not be given to patients with anaemia secondary to vitamin B_{12} deficiency and folate as this may precipitate subacute combined degeneration of the spinal cord. In this case it should be administered in conjunction with vitamin B_{12}.

Interactions
*   No significant interactions.

Route of administration
*   Oral.

Note
*   The cause of folate deficiency should be ascertained and corrected prior to folate therapy.
*   Folate is absorbed in the proximal jejunum. Folate deficiency is therefore a leading finding in coeliac disease.
*   In order to prevent fetal neural tube defects, women should be started on daily folic acid supplements 4 weeks prior to conception and should continue until the 12th week of pregnancy. Higher doses are needed if patient on antiepileptic medication or has a family history of neural tube defects.

HISTAMINE$_2$ (H$_2$) ANTAGONISTS

(Cimetidine, famotidine, nizatidine, ranitidine)

Class: H$_2$ antagonist

Indications
* Gastro-oesophageal reflux disease.
* Prophylaxis of NSAID-associated gastric or duodenal ulcers.
* Treatment of duodenal and gastric ulcers.

Mechanism of action
* These drugs decrease gastric acid production by blocking the effect of histamine on parietal cells in the stomach. They act as competitive antagonists at membrane-bound H$_2$ receptors on parietal cells which produce acid.
* Maximum therapeutic response is achieved in the fasting state.

Adverse effects
* *Common*: diarrhoea, rash.
* *Rare*: acute pancreatitis, cardiac dysrhythmias, confusion, alopecia, erythema multiforme, deranged LFTs.

Contraindications
* None.

Interactions
* No significant interactions except with cimetidine, an enzyme inhibitor that can potentiate action of other drugs. Cimetidine is rarely used nowadays.

Route of administration
* Oral, IM, IV.

Note
* Ranitidine should heal roughly 90% of duodenal ulcers after 8 weeks of therapy. It can also be used to treat gastric ulcers; however, PPIs (e.g. omeprazole) are preferred in clinical practice.
* Gastric cancer must be excluded before prescribing ranitidine to elderly and middle-aged patients as it may mask the symptoms and thus delay diagnosis.
* Ranitidine is preferred to cimetidine because it has fewer adverse effects and fewer drug interactions. Unlike cimetidine, it does not cause impotence in young men and does not cause confusion in the elderly.
* H$_2$-receptor antagonists are of no use in the management of acute upper GI haemorrhage.
* Unlike cimetidine, ranitidine is not a hepatic enzyme inhibitor.

HYDROXOCOBALAMIN

Class: Vitamin B_{12}

Indications
* Pernicious anaemia.
* Other vitamin B_{12}-deficiency states (e.g. following gastrectomy or ileal resection).
* Leber's optic atrophy.
* Schilling test.

Mechanism of action
* Hydroxocobalamin is needed for synthesis of purines and pyrimidines and their subsequent incorporation into DNA.

Adverse effects
* *Rare*: anaphylaxis, nausea, dizziness, pruritus, fever.

Contraindications
* None.

Interactions
* None.

Route of administration
* IM.

Note
* Hydroxocobalamin has replaced oral cyanocobalamin as therapeutic vitamin B_{12} because it is retained in the body for a longer period of time.
* Dietary vitamin B_{12} is absorbed in the terminal ileum.
* Schilling test was employed in the diagnosis of pernicious anaemia but is rarely used nowadays.
* Hydroxocobalamin injections are given on alternate days for the first 2 weeks and once every 3 months thereafter as maintenance therapy (usually for life).
* It takes approximately 2 years for the body's vitamin B_{12} stores to become depleted.

LACTULOSE

Class: Osmotic laxative

Indications
*   Constipation.
*   Hepatic encephalopathy in liver disease.

Mechanism of action
*   Lactulose is a disaccharide consisting of fructose and galactose.
*   Lactulose stimulates bowel peristalsis by increasing the volume of intestinal contents. It cannot be metabolized by human disaccharidases and reaches the colon virtually unchanged, where it is hydrolysed by bacteria into simple organic acids (mainly lactic acid). These components draw water into the lumen of the large bowel by osmosis.
*   Lactulose also decreases the pH of gut contents, thus reducing the activity of ammonia-producing organisms, hence its use in hepatic encephalopathy (ammonia is thought to cross the blood–brain barrier and act as a false neurotransmitter, thus causing the symptoms of hepatic encephalopathy).

Adverse effects
*   *Common*: flatulence, abdominal cramps, diarrhoea.
*   *Rare*: nausea, vomiting.

Contraindications
*   Intestinal obstruction.
*   Galactosaemia.

Interactions
*   None (as it is not absorbed).

Route of administration
*   Oral.

Note
*   Lactulose can take up to 48 hours to have an effect.
*   It can be given to prevent constipation caused by opioid analgesics.
*   Dose is gradually increased until patient is satisfied with their bowel frequency and stool consistency.

Related drugs
*   Macrogols, magnesium salts, phosphate enema, sodium citrate enema.

LOPERAMIDE

Class: Opioid antimotility drug

Indications
*   Symptomatic management of acute diarrhoea.
*   Supplement to rehydration in acute diarrhoea (patients over
4 years of age only).
*   Chronic diarrhoea (adults only) for symptomatic relief, e.g.
irritable bowel syndrome.

Mechanism of action
*   Loperamide acts on opioid mu receptors in the myenteric plexus
of the gut wall. It inhibits acetylcholine release from the myenteric
plexus and hence inhibits peristalsis.
*   It also increases the tone of the anal sphincter.

Adverse effects
*   *Common*: abdominal cramps.
*   *Rare*: constipation, abdominal bloating, rash, paralytic ileus.

Contraindications
*   Active inflammatory bowel disease.
*   Antibiotic-associated colitis.
*   Infective diarrhoea.

Interactions
*   None.

Route of administration
*   Oral.

Note
*   Loperamide should not be used for long periods of time. Further
investigation into the cause of diarrhoea should be undertaken if no
improvement is seen after a few days of treatment.
*   Unlike other opioids, loperamide does not easily penetrate the
blood–brain barrier, which makes it unlikely to cause central effects
and dependence.

Related drugs
*   Codeine phosphate, co-phenotrope.

METOCLOPRAMIDE

Class: Dopamine$_2$ (D$_2$) antagonist

Indications
* Nausea and vomiting (due to drugs, chemotherapy, radiotherapy, migraine).
* Gastro-oesophageal reflux disease.
* Barium follow-through investigation.
* Oesophageal dysmotility disorder.

Mechanism of action
* Metoclopramide has several actions, all of which contribute to its antiemetic effect:
    1. It blocks D$_2$ receptors in the chemoreceptor trigger zone in the brainstem.
    2. It increases the rate of gastric and duodenal emptying by causing relaxation of the pyloric sphincter. It also increases lower oesophageal sphincter tone and oesophageal motility helping in gastro-oesophageal reflux disease.
* In barium follow-through, metoclopramide speeds up barium transit.

Adverse effects
* *Rare*: tardive dyskinesia, neuroleptic malignant syndrome, hyperprolactinaemia, depression, cardiac conduction abnormalities, diarrhoea, acute dystonic reactions (e.g. oculogyric crisis).

Contraindications
* Intestinal obstruction, haemorrhage or perforation.
* The first 3–4 days following GI surgery.
* Breastfeeding.
* Phaeochromocytoma.

Interactions
* *Analgesics*: metoclopramide increases the absorption of paracetamol and aspirin, thus enhancing their effects.
* *Antipsychotics*: metoclopramide increases the risk of extrapyramidal adverse effects.

Route of administration
* Oral, IM, IV.

Note
* Nausea and vomiting in migraine can cause gastric stasis, which reduces the absorption rate of aspirin and paracetamol. In order to accelerate their absorption, aspirin and paracetamol can be combined with metoclopramide.
* Acute dystonic reactions are more common in young females of child-bearing age taking metoclopramide. These can be treated with an anticholinergic benzatropine or procyclidine.
* Metoclopramide is not effective against motion sickness.
* Domperidone has similar pharmacological actions to metoclopramide, but is less likely to cause CNS effects due to its poor transport across the blood–brain barrier.

Related drugs
* Domperidone.

ONDANSETRON

Class: Serotonin (5-hydroxytryptamine [5-HT$_3$]) antagonist

Indications
- Treatment and prophylaxis of nausea and vomiting (in chemotherapy, radiotherapy and postoperatively).

Mechanism of action
- Exact mechanism is not fully understood.
- Ondansetron selectively blocks excitatory serotonin receptors in the chemoreceptor trigger zone of the brain and in the GI tract.

Adverse effects
- *Common*: headache, constipation, flushing.
- *Rare*: deranged LFTs, transient visual disturbances, seizures.

Contraindications
- None
- Caution:
  - Pregnancy.
  - Breastfeeding.
  - Hepatic impairment.

Interactions
- None.

Route of administration
- Oral, IM, IV, rectal.

Note
- The effect of ondansetron can be enhanced by adding a single dose of dexamethasone in the treatment of chemotherapy-induced nausea and vomiting.

Related drugs
- Dolasetron, granisetron, palonosetron, tropisetron.

PANCREATIN

Class: Enzyme-containing pancreas extract

Indications
- Reduced or absent pancreatic exocrine secretions (e.g. in cystic fibrosis, chronic pancreatitis, following pancreatectomy).

Mechanism of action
- Pancreatin contains protease for breakdown of proteins, amylase for breakdown of starch and lipase for breakdown of fats.
- These enzymes are essential for an efficient digestive process.

Adverse effects
- *Common*: nausea, vomiting, diarrhoea, abdominal discomfort.
- *Rare*: hypersensitivity, perianal irritation (with excessive doses).

Contraindications
- None.

Interactions
- No significant interactions.

Route of administration
- Oral.

Note
- Pancreatin should be taken with food. Additionally, H_2-receptor antagonists (e.g. ranitidine) or antacids can be given in conjunction with pancreatin to prevent destruction of the pancreatic enzymes by gastric acid.
- Excessive heat inactivates the enzymes contained in pancreatin. It should therefore not be mixed with hot foods or hot liquids.
- Enteric-coated preparations carry more of the enzymes to the duodenum. This makes pancreatin therapy more efficient.

PEGINTERFERON ALFA AND INTERFERON ALFA

Class: Antiviral

Indications
* Treatment of chronic hepatitis C infection.
* Treatment of chronic hepatitis B infection.

Mechanism of action
* Binds to cell-surface receptors leading to a cascade of interactions that activate certain genes. This leads to inhibition of viral replication and immunomodulatory effects.

Adverse effects
* *Common*: flu-like symptoms, myelosuppresion, psychiatric illness.
* *Rare*: alopecia, hepatitis, renal impairment, cardiovascular effects (hypotension, hypertension, arrhythmias).

Contraindications
* Severe depression.
* Pregnancy and breastfeeding.
* Decompensated cirrhosis.
* Autoimmune disease.

Interactions
* Theophylline: interferons lead to increased levels of theophylline.

Route of administration
* SC – peginterferon alfa.
* IV – interferon alfa.

Note
* If there is haematological toxicity, depression, renal or hepatic impairment, the dose of interferons should be reduced. If adverse effects persist or worsen, consider stopping therapy.
* Myelosuppresion is not uncommon and may require supportive treatment with erythropoietin (EPO) injections and granulocyte-colony stimulating factor (G-CSF) treatment. Sometimes transfusion of blood products may be required.
* Blood monitoring weekly for 3 weeks and then monthly is recommended.
* Interferons can trigger autoimmune diseases hence wise to check thyroid function regularly and monitor for symptoms.
* Flu-like symptoms usually occur 6–8 hours post dose.

PROTON PUMP INHIBITORS (PPIs)

(Esomeprazole, lansoprazole, omeprazole, pantoprazole, rabeprazole,)

Class: Proton pump inhibitor (PPI)

Indications
- Prophylaxis and treatment of gastric or duodenal ulcers.
- Part of *Helicobacter pylori* eradication therapy in combination with antibiotics.
- Gastro-oesophageal reflux disease, oesophagitis, Barrett's oesophagus, gastritis.
- Zollinger–Ellison syndrome.

Mechanism of action
- These drugs cause dose-dependent irreversible inhibition of gastric acid production by inhibiting the H^+/K^+ ATPase ('proton pump') in gastric parietal cells. Acid secretion is thus inhibited by over 90%.

Adverse effects
- *Common*: headache, diarrhoea, rash.
- *Rare*: Stevens–Johnson syndrome, gynaecomastia, hypersensitivity reactions, hepatic or renal impairment, blurred vision, haematological disorders (e.g. pancytopenia, thrombocytopenia).

Contraindications
- None.

Interactions
- *Phenytoin*: omeprazole increases the plasma concentration of phenytoin.
- *Warfarin*: omeprazole increases the plasma concentration of warfarin.
- *Note*: Omeprazole inhibits hepatic drug-metabolizing enzymes, hence a wide range of further interactions exists.

Route of administration
- Oral, IV.

Note
- Pantoprazole and rabeprazole have the least drug interactions.
- PPIs may mask the symptoms of a gastric or oesophageal cancer, therefore it is important to exclude malignancy prior to treatment in individuals over 45 years old with new symptoms, or in anyone with alarm symptoms, e.g. dysphagia, weight loss, bleeding.
- Esomeprazole is usually reserved for severe cases.
- PPIs reduce re-bleeding rate and endoscopic therapy if given before endoscopy in an acute upper GI bleed.
- There has been some recent controversy about the combination of a PPI and clopidogrel leading to an increased risk of cardiac events but further studies are required before recommendations can be made.

RIBAVIRIN

Class: Antiviral

Indications
* Treatment of hepatitis C infection – in conjunction with peginterferon alfa or interferon alfa.
* Treatment of respiratory syncytial virus bronchiolitis in children.

Mechanism of action
* Ribavirin is a prodrug that interferes with RNA and DNA metabolism required for viral replication.

Adverse effects
* *Common*: haemolytic anaemia.
* *Rare*: depression, psychiatric illness.

Contraindications
* Pregnancy and breastfeeding.
* Men whose female partners are pregnant (unless use condom).
* Haemoglobinopathies (sickle cell, thalassaemia).
* Decompensated cirrhosis.
* Uncontrolled severe depression.
* Autoimmune disease.
* Severe cardiac failure.

Interactions
* Nil significant.

Route of administration
* Oral, nebulizer for bronchiolitis.

Note
* Exclude pregnancy before treatment because ribavirin is very teratogenic.
* Not to be given to females during pregnancy or within 4 months of planned pregnancy.
* Males receiving ribavirin should use condoms during, and for 6 months after, treatment and when their female partners are pregnant.
* Patients with severe cardiac disease should not be given ribavirin, as the drug-induced haemolytic anaemia can cause decompensation of cardiac disease.
* Only use ribavirin with interferon as it is ineffective as monotherapy in the treatment of hepatitis C infection.

SENNA

Class: Stimulant laxative

Indications
* Constipation.

Mechanism of action
* Senna is hydrolysed by bacteria in the colon to produce anthracene glycoside derivatives that are irritant to the GI tract. These stimulate the myenteric (Auerbach's) plexus in the gut wall to increase peristalsis.

Adverse effects
* *Common*: abdominal cramps, diarrhoea.
* *Rare*: hypokalaemia, colonic atony (with prolonged use).

Contraindications
* Intestinal obstruction.

Interactions
* None.

Route of administration
* Oral.

Note
* Senna acts within 8–12 hours.
* Regular use of senna can lead to tolerance and should therefore be used for short periods only.
* Patients taking senna should be warned about the dangers of continuous use (e.g. hypokalaemia, atonic colon).
* A high-fibre intake (e.g. fruit, vegetable, whole wheat) should be encouraged.

Related drugs
* Bisacodyl, dantron, docusate sodium, glycerol suppository, sodium picosulphate.

URSODEOXYCHOLIC ACID

Class: Bile acid

Indications
* Treatment of primary biliary cirrhosis.
* Treatment of primary sclerosing cholangitis.
* Dissolution of small–medium cholesterol-rich gallstones.

Mechanism of action
* Ursodeoxycholic acid improves elevated liver enzymes by facilitating bile flow through the liver.
* Reduces cholesterol absorption from the intestine and dissolves cholesterol gallstones.

Adverse effects
* *Rare*: diarrhoea, vomiting, nausea, pruritus, gallstone calcification (preventing dissolution).

Contraindications
* Radio-opaque stones.
* Pregnancy.
* Non-functioning gallbladder.
* GI conditions that interfere with enterohepatic circulation of bile salts.

Interactions
* *Ciclosporin*: ursodeoxycholic acid increases absorption of ciclosporin.
* *COC pill, lipid-lowering drugs*: these can reduce effectiveness of therapy by lowering blood cholesterol and thereby increasing bile cholesterol levels.

Route of administration
* Oral.

Note
* In primary biliary cirrhosis and primary sclerosing cholangitis ursodeoxycholic acid improves liver biochemistry but there is ongoing debate as to whether it improves the natural history of these conditions.
* Effective for small to medium (up to 10 mm) radiolucent stones (mainly cholesterol) in those with a functioning gallbladder. Duration of therapy can be 6–18 months and radiological monitoring is required.
* Cholesterol stones coated with calcium and bile pigment stones are not dissolved by ursodeoxycholic acid.

NEUROLOGICAL SYSTEM

Management guidelines (pp. 81–84)
Epilepsy
Migraine
Idiopathic Parkinson's disease
Stroke

Drugs (pp. 85–94)
Bromocriptine
Carbamazepine
Diazepam
Dipyridamole
Gabapentin
Levetiracetam
Levodopa
Phenytoin
Sodium valproate
Sumatriptan

Management guidelines

EPILEPSY
* Treatment should be tailored to the individual and use monotherapy whenever possible.
* The following factors should be taken into consideration before commencing therapy: seizure type, epilepsy syndrome, co-morbidities, co-medication, lifestyle and preferences of the individual.
* In some individuals, combination therapy with two or more antiepileptic drugs is required to reduce seizure frequency; used when monotherapy with two different drugs fails or seizures occur on monotherapy when maximum-tolerated dose used.
* Psychological interventions and vagal nerve stimulators can be used as adjunctive therapy when there is inadequate seizure control with optimal antiepileptic drugs.
* Older antiepileptic drugs: benzodiazepines (clobazam, clonazepam), carbamazepine, phenytoin, barbiturates (phenobarbital, primidone), sodium valproate.
* Newer antiepileptic drugs: gabapentin, lamotrigine, levetiracetam, oxcarbazepine, pregabalin, tiagabine, topiramate, vigabatrin.

The Hands–on Guide to Clinical Pharmacology, 3rd Edition. By S Chatu.
Published 2010 by Blackwell Publishing Ltd.

- Carbamazepine, oxcarbazepine, phenytoin and phenobarbital are hepatic enzyme inducing drugs, e.g. can reduce the effectiveness of the COC pill.
- The choice of drug depends on the seizure type or epilepsy syndrome, how well it is tolerated and factors mentioned above.

Partial seizures with or without secondary generalization
- First-line choices: carbamazepine, lamotrigine, oxcarbazepine, sodium valproate, topiramate.
- Second-line choices: clobazam, gabapentin, levetiracetam, pregabalin, tiagabine.

Generalized seizures
Tonic–clonic
- First-line choices: carbamazepine, lamotrigine, sodium valproate, topiramate.
- Second-line choices: clobazam, levetiracetam, oxcarbazepine.

Absence seizures
- First-line choices: ethosuximide, sodium valproate.
- Second-line choices: clonazepam, lamotrigine.

Myoclonic seizures
- First-line choices: sodium valproate.
- Second-line choices: clonazepam, lamotrigine, levetiracetam, topiramate.

Atonic and tonic seizures
- First-line choices: clonazepam, lamotrigine, sodium valproate.
- Second-line choices: clobazam, ethosuximide, levetiracetam, topiramate.

Status epilepticus
- This is a seizure lasting longer than 30 minutes, or recurrent seizures without gaining consciousness.
- Give oxygen through face mask and position patient to avoid injury and consider airway adjuncts.
- Give IV lorazepam or diazepam (rectal diazepam or buccal midazolam if IV access not possible).
- If seizures reoccur, repeat lorazepam or diazepam.
- Give IV thiamine if alcohol is thought to be involved.
- Give 50 ml of 50% dextrose IV if blood glucose is low.
- If seizure persists, add IV phenytoin (attach cardiac monitor to detect any dysrhythmias and hypotension induced by phenytoin).
- If still fitting, consider IV phenobarbitone, get expert help and consider mechanical ventilation under general anaesthesia using propofol, thiopentone or a midazolam infusion.
- Once stable, start oral antiepileptic drugs and investigate to find cause, e.g. non-compliance with antiepileptic medication or infection, and treat appropriately.

MIGRAINE
Acute attacks
- Give paracetamol, or soluble aspirin or other NSAIDs (e.g. diclofenac, ibuprofen).

- Metoclopramide can be given for associated nausea and vomiting (and also to increase the rate of absorption of aspirin and paracetamol).
- Give a triptan, e.g. sumatriptan (a 5-HT$_1$ agonist) if the above fails. This can be given orally, as intranasal spray or SC.
- In refractory cases, corticosteroids may be used.
- Ergotamine, an alpha agonist, is rarely used but may be tried if all else fails (contraindicated in ischaemic heart disease).

Prophylaxis
- Prophylaxis is given to patients who experience more than one severe migraine attack per month.
- Avoid precipitating factors (mainly emotional factors but also chocolate, cheese, alcohol, lack of sleep, COC pill).
- The following drugs can be tried: oral pizotifen (a 5-HT$_2$ antagonist), oral propranolol or amitriptyline.
- Sodium valproate, carbamazepine, verapamil, topiramate and gabapentin are alternatives that may be tried if above measures fail.
- The prophylactic medication is usually changed if no benefit after 3 months.

IDIOPATHIC PARKINSON'S DISEASE
Supportive treatment
- Regular access to specialist nursing care.
- Physiotherapy may be helpful in maintaining joint and muscle mobility and ensuring independence.
- Involve the occupational therapist, social worker and speech therapist.
- In advanced disease, involve palliative care services.
- Important to manage other associated problems that occur in Parkinson's disease, such as depression, dementia, psychotic symptoms, falls, sleep disturbance and constipation.

Pharmacological treatment
- Anti-Parkinsonian drugs improve quality of life by alleviating symptoms, but they do not prevent progression of the disease.
- Treatment of choice: levodopa with a peripheral decarboxylase inhibitor (benserazide or carbidopa).
- Other options are dopamine agonists, antimuscarinics and other drugs.

Dopamine agonists
- These are reserved for cases where levodopa is no longer effective or no longer tolerated.
- They are also used in younger patients with early Parkinson's disease.
- Dopamine agonists include ergot derived (bromocriptine, cabergoline, pergolide) and non-ergot derived (apomorphine, pramipexole, ropinirole, rotigine).
- The ergot-derived dopamine agonists are associated with pulmonary, pericardial and retroperitoneal fibrosis, hence the non-ergot derived are preferred.

Antimuscarinics

- These counteract the cholinergic excess that is believed to occur in Parkinson's disease.
- They are used in drug-induced Parkinsonism or if tremor is a prominent symptom.
- They include benzatropine, orphenadrine, procyclidine and trihexyphenidyl.

Other drugs

- Monoamine oxidase (MAO) type B inhibitors selegiline and rasagiline can be used early in the disease process or combined with levodopa in advanced Parkinson's disease.
- Catechyl-O-methyl transferase (COMT) inhibitors: entacapone and tolcapone prevent peripheral breakdown of levodopa by inhibiting the enzyme COMT, thus allowing more levodopa to reach the brain. Sometimes used in late Parkinson's disease as an adjunct to levodopa preparations.
- Risk of neuroleptic malignant syndrome and acute akinesia if antiparkinsonism medication is withdrawn suddenly.
- Dopamine dysregulation syndrome is something to be aware of in patients on treatment. This condition leads to abnormal behaviour, e.g. gambling, hypersexuality.
- Sudden onset of sleep and excessive sleepiness can occur with levodopa preparations and dopamine agonists so it is important to warn patients about this.

Surgery

- Thalamic stimulators for severe tremor unresponsive to medical therapy.
- Bilateral deep brain stimulators for suitable patients that do not respond to medical therapy.

STROKE

- All patients with a suspected stroke should be admitted to a stroke unit.
- Patients presenting within 3 hours of onset of symptoms with a confirmed ischaemic stroke on imaging should be considered for thrombolysis, providing they meet certain criteria.
- Aspirin and dipyridamole should be started in ischaemic stroke (if unable to swallow give aspirin alone via rectal enema or administer both drugs via nasogastric tube).
- Supportive management is required in haemorrhagic stroke; however, neurosurgical intervention may be required if hydrocephalus develops.
- On admission, screen swallow before giving any oral fluid, food or medication.
- If swallow is impaired, start IV fluids and refer for specialist assessment with view to starting a modified diet or enteral feeding with regular review.
- Initiate nutritional support if patient is malnourished.
- Involvement of the multidisciplinary stroke team in providing stroke rehabilitation is of the upmost importance with modification of risk factors to prevent further events.

Drugs

BROMOCRIPTINE

Class: Dopamine agonist

Indications
- Idiopathic Parkinson's disease.
- Hyperprolactinaemia.
- Acromegaly.
- Cyclical benign breast disease.
- Prevention and suppression of lactation.

Mechanism of action
- Bromocriptine stimulates D_2 receptors in the CNS. This accounts for its use in Parkinson's disease.
- Bromocriptine is useful in hyperprolactinaemia as it inhibits the release of prolactin from the anterior pituitary gland. This inhibits lactation. Bromocriptine also reduces the size of prolactinomas.
- Bromocriptine inhibits the release of growth hormone in acromegaly. Note: in unaffected individuals growth hormone levels are *raised* by bromocriptine.

Adverse effects
- *Common*: nausea, vomiting, constipation, postural hypotension, headache.
- *Rare*: confusion, drowsiness, dyskinesia, vasospasm in fingers and toes, pulmonary, pericardial or retroperitoneal fibrosis.

Contraindications
- Pre-eclampsia.
- Postpartum hypertension.

Interactions
- *Erythromycin*: increases the plasma concentration of bromocriptine, thus increasing the risk of dose-dependent adverse effects.

Route of administration
- Oral.

Note
- High doses of bromocriptine are normally used in the treatment of acromegaly and Parkinson's disease. This leads to a higher incidence of adverse effects.
- Nausea and vomiting can be decreased by increasing the dose of bromocriptine slowly and taking it with meals.
- Domperidone can be used to reduce the systemic adverse effects of bromocriptine. It does not reduce central adverse effects as it does not cross the blood–brain barrier.
- Sudden onset of sleep and excessive sleepiness can occur with dopamine agonists so it is important to warn patients about this.
- Monitor for symptoms suggestive of fibrotic reactions, e.g. breathlessness, cough, abdominal pain.

Related drugs
- Cabergoline, pergolide, quinagolide.

CARBAMAZEPINE

Class: Anticonvulsant

Indications
- Generalized tonic–clonic seizures.
- Partial seizures.
- Trigeminal neuralgia and other chronic neuropathic pain.
- Prophylaxis of bipolar disorder.

Mechanism of action
- Exact mechanism is not fully understood.
- Carbamazepine is thought to:
  1. Enhance gamma-aminobutyric acid (GABA)-mediated inhibitory transmission in the CNS.
  2. Decrease electrical excitability of neuronal cell membranes by blocking sodium and calcium channels.

Adverse effects
- *Common*: rash, in elderly – drowsiness, blurred vision, confusion.
- *Rare*: agranulocytosis, thrombocytopenia, hepatic failure, acute renal failure, cardiac conduction abnormalities, osteomalacia, hyponatraemia, ataxia, Stevens–Johnson syndrome, toxic epidermal necrolysis.

Contraindications
- Bone marrow suppression.
- AV node conduction abnormalities (unless pacemaker *in situ*).
- Acute porphyria.

Interactions
- *Diltiazem, erythromycin, verapamil*: increase the plasma concentration of carbamazepine.
- *COC pill*: carbamazepine reduces the effect of oral contraceptives.
- *Warfarin*: carbamazepine reduces the effect of warfarin.
- *Note*: carbamazepine induces hepatic drug-metabolizing enzymes, hence a wide range of further interactions exists.

Route of administration
- Oral, rectal (for epilepsy, if oral route not possible).

Note
- It is important to start therapy with a low dose in order to minimize adverse effects. The dose is then increased in small increments every 2 weeks until symptoms are controlled.
- It is recommended to monitor the FBC, LFTs and renal function while on carbamazepine therapy.
- Carbamazepine can cause folate deficiency. It may cause neural tube defects or hypospadias in the fetus.
- Carbamazepine can induce its own metabolism and also causes hyponatraemia due to syndrome of inappropriate antidiuretic hormone (SIADH) secretion.
- Serious skin reactions are more common in those with ancestry from Asia who have the HLA-B1502 allele.

Related drugs
- Oxcarbazepine.

DIAZEPAM

Class: Benzodiazepine

Indications
- Short term use in anxiety states and insomnia.
- Status epilepticus.
- Febrile convulsions.
- Muscle spasm (e.g. spasticity).

Mechanism of action
- Diazepam facilitates opening of chloride channels in the CNS by binding to the GABA/chloride-channel complex. The resulting flow of chloride ions results in hyperpolarization and therefore neuronal inhibition. It is thought that this action produces the anxiolytic, anticonvulsant and sedative effects.

Adverse effects
- *Common*: daytime drowsiness, confusion in the elderly.
- *Rare*: headache, blurred vision, confusion, rash, thrombophlebitis (with IV injection), respiratory depression, apnoea.

Contraindications
- Respiratory depression.
- Sleep apnoea syndrome.
- Severe hepatic impairment.
- Neuromuscular weakness, e.g. myasthenia gravis, motor neuron disease.

Interactions
- *Isoniazid*: inhibits the metabolism of diazepam.
- *Rifampicin*: increases the metabolism of diazepam.
- *Sedatives*: enhance the sedative effect of diazepam.

Route of administration
- Oral, rectal (if oral route inappropriate), IM or IV (status epilepticus, acute severe anxiety).

Note
- Diazepam is metabolized by the liver to active metabolites that have very long half-lives (e.g. *N*-desmethyldiazepam has a half-life of up to 200 hours). Accumulation of active metabolites can therefore easily occur.
- Midazolam is used to provide short-acting sedation prior to certain procedures, e.g. endoscopy, shoulder manipulation.
- Flurazepam, nitrazepam and temazepam are used in the short-term treatment of insomnia.
- Flumazenil is a specific benzodiazepine antagonist that can be given in benzodiazepine overdose, but may precipitate a withdrawal syndrome.
- Clobazam and clonazepam are used in the treatment of epilepsy.
- Chlordiazepoxide is used in the treatment of alcohol detoxification.

Related drugs
- Alprazolam, chlordiazepoxide, clobazam, clonazepam, flurazepam, lorazepam, midazolam, nitrazepam, oxazepam.

DIPYRIDAMOLE

Class: Antithrombotic

Indications
* Secondary prophylaxis of ischaemic stroke.
* Transient ischaemic attack (TIA).

Mechanism of action
* Inhibit platelet aggregation by preventing adenosine uptake into platelets. Dipyridamole also increases cAMP concentration in platelets by inhibiting phosphodiesterase, which leads to low intracellular calcium levels thereby inhibiting platelet activation and granule release.

Adverse effects
* *Common*: headache, dizziness, nausea, vomiting, diarrhoea.
* *Rare*: hepatitis, worsening symptoms of IHD, hypotension, tachycardia hypersensitivity reactions, e.g. bronchospasm, rash.

Contraindications
* Nil.

Interactions
* *Adenosine*: dipyridamole enhances and prolongs the effects of adenosine.
* *Heparin, warfarin*: anticoagulant effect is enhanced.
* *Clopidogrel*: increased risk of bleeding.

Route of administration
* Oral.

Note
* Adverse effects are usually minimal and transient but in those who do not tolerate dipyridamole the dose should be increased gradually.
* After an ischaemic stroke or TIA, aspirin should be used in combination with dipyridamole for a period of 2 years with continuation of aspirin alone thereafter.
* There is a combination product available containing aspirin and dipyridamole.
* Dipyridamole should be avoided in those with myasthenia gravis as it may precipitate a crisis.

GABAPENTIN

Class: Anticonvulsant

Indications
*   Treatment of partial seizures with or without secondary generalization.
*   Chronic neuropathic pain, e.g. post-herpetic neuralgia, diabetic neuropathy, trigeminal neuralgia.

Mechanism of action
*   Exact mechanism is unknown.
*   Has an analgesic and anticonvulsant effect.

Adverse effects
*   *Common*: dizziness, drowsiness, peripheral oedema, GI symptoms.
*   *Rare*: fatigue, neurological signs and symptoms, hepatitis, pancreatitis.

Contraindications
*   Pregnancy (use only if benefits outweigh risks to the fetus after specialist advice).
*   Breastfeeding.

Interactions
*   *TCAs, SSRIs, MAOIs*: these antidepressants antagonize the anticonvulsant effect of gabapentin.

Route of administration
*   Oral, IV.

Note
*   Antiepileptic drugs have been associated with an increased risk of suicidal behaviour/thinking, so patients should be closely monitored and appropriate action taken.
*   Dose should be reduced in renal impairment.
*   Abrupt withdrawal of gabapentin can lead to a withdrawal syndrome.
*   Gabapentin can cause a false-positive reaction with certain urine dipstick tests when testing for urinary protein.
*   Pregabalin is a similar drug which is also used in the treatment of epilepsy, neuropathic pain and generalized anxiety disorder.

LEVETIRACETAM

Class: Anticonvulsant

Indications
* Monotherapy and adjunctive treatment of epilepsy.

Mechanism of action
* Exact mechanism is unknown.
* Inhibits spread of seizure activity in the brain.
* Animal studies have shown drug to act on synapses and impair nerve conduction.

Adverse effects
* *Common*: sleepiness, tiredness, headache, infections (nasopharyngitis).
* *Rare*: leucopenia, dizziness, ataxia, depression, tremor, psychiatric symptoms.

Contraindications
* Pregnancy (use only if benefits outweigh risks to the fetus after specialist advice).
* Breastfeeding.

Interactions
* *Probenecid*: reduces elimination of levetiracetam.

Route of administration
* Oral, IV.

Note
* Antiepileptic drugs have been associated with an increased risk of suicidal behaviour/thinking, so patients should be closely monitored and appropriate action taken.
* Dose should be reduced in renal impairment.

LEVODOPA

Class: Dopamine precursor

Indications
- Idiopathic Parkinson's disease.

Mechanism of action
- Levodopa is an amino acid precursor of dopamine. It crosses the blood–brain barrier and is then converted to dopamine by the enzyme dopa decarboxylase. This action replaces dopamine, which is deficient in the basal ganglia in Parkinson's disease. Dopamine itself is not used in Parkinson's disease as it cannot cross the blood–brain barrier.

Adverse effects
- Common:
    - Systemic adverse effects – nausea, vomiting, abdominal pain, anorexia, postural hypotension, dizziness, discoloration of urine and other body fluids.
    - CNS adverse effects – abnormal involuntary movements, 'on–off effect' (rigidity alternating with excessive movements).
- Rare: psychiatric symptoms (e.g. confusion, hallucinations, depression), cardiac dysrhythmias.

Contraindications
- Closed-angle glaucoma.
- Drug-induced Parkinsonism.

Interactions
- *Anaesthetics*: concomitant use of levodopa and volatile liquid anaesthetics increases the risk of cardiac dysrhythmias.
- *MAOIs*: risk of hypertensive crisis (withdraw MAOIs 2 weeks before starting levodopa).
- *Neuroleptics*: these reduce the effects of levodopa by blocking dopamine receptors.

Route of administration
- Oral.

Note
- Only low levels of levodopa reach the brain as it is peripherally converted to dopamine by dopa decarboxylase. Combining levodopa with a decarboxylase inhibitor, such as benserazide or carbidopa, can prevent this. Thus, more dopamine reaches the brain and a reduction in systemic adverse effects is achieved.
- The efficacy of levodopa decreases with long-term use.
- Anticholinergic drugs (e.g. benzhexol) may be helpful in controlling tremor and excess salivation that occur in Parkinson's disease.

PHENYTOIN

Class: Anticonvulsant

Indications
* All types of epilepsy, except absence seizures.
* Status epilepticus.
* Trigeminal neuralgia.

Mechanism of action
* Phenytoin alters transmembrane movement of Na^+ and K^+ by blocking voltage-gated Na^+ channels. This action stabilizes neuronal thresholds against hyperexcitability.
* Phenytoin acts primarily in the motor cortex of the brain. It is thought to prevent the spread of epileptic discharges, not the initiation.

Adverse effects
* *Common*: dizziness, insomnia, nausea, vomiting, coarsening of facial features, hirsutism, acne.
* *Rare*: gum hypertrophy, Stevens–Johnson syndrome, drug-induced systemic lupus erythematosus (SLE), peripheral neuropathy, Dupuytren's contracture, hepatitis, cardiac dysrhythmias, folic acid and vitamin D deficiency.

Contraindications
* None.
* Caution:
  * Pregnancy and breastfeeding.

Interactions
* *Amiodarone, cimetidine, diltiazem*: these drugs increase the plasma concentration of phenytoin.
* *COC pill*: phenytoin decreases the effect of the COC pill by increasing its metabolism.
* *Warfarin*: phenytoin increases the metabolism of warfarin.
* *Note*: phenytoin induces hepatic drug-metabolizing enzymes hence a wide range of further interactions exists.

Route of administration
* Oral (epilepsy, trigeminal neuralgia), IV (epilepsy).

Note
* Phenytoin has a narrow therapeutic window and a non-linear relationship between dose and plasma concentration (zero-order kinetics). It therefore requires therapeutic drug monitoring.
* Patients should be advised how to recognize signs of phenytoin toxicity (mostly CNS effects: tremor, nystagmus, ataxia, dysarthria and convulsions).
* Owing to cosmetic adverse effects, phenytoin may be undesirable for use in adolescents.
* Phenytoin is teratogenic and is associated with congenital heart disease and cleft palate/lip. Antenatal screening is recommended.
* If phenytoin is given IV, cardiac monitoring is essential (risk of dysrhythmias and hypotension).
* Nowadays, phenytoin is mainly used in the treatment of status epilepticus. Its adverse effects limit long-term use in epilepsy.

Related drugs
* Fosphenytoin (a prodrug of phenytoin).

SODIUM VALPROATE

Class: Anticonvulsant

Indications
- All types of epilepsy.
- Migraine prophylaxis.
- Chronic neuropathic pain.

Mechanism of action
- Sodium valproate increases GABA content of the brain by inhibiting the enzyme GABA transaminase and preventing GABA re-uptake.
- Sodium valproate also reduces concentrations of aspartate, an excitatory neurotransmitter.
- In addition, it blocks voltage-gated sodium channels.

Adverse effects
- *Common*: nausea, vomiting, weight gain.
- *Rare*: hepatic failure, pancreatitis, blood dyscrasias (pancytopenia, thrombocytopenia, leucopenia), sedation, transient hair loss, hyponatraemia, Stevens–Johnson syndrome.

Contraindications
- Acute liver failure (sodium valproate is metabolized and excreted by the liver).
- Acute porphyria.

Interactions
- *Anticonvulsants*: two or more anticonvulsants given together may lead to enhanced effects, increased sedation or reduced plasma concentrations of either drug.
- *Neuroleptics*: decrease the anticonvulsant effect of sodium valproate.
- *TCAs*: decrease the anticonvulsant effect of sodium valproate.

Route of administration
- Oral, IV.

Note
- LFTs should be monitored during therapy, particularly in the first 6 months of treatment.
- Sodium valproate is especially useful in children with atonic epilepsy or absence seizures as it has little sedative effect.
- Sodium valproate has fewer adverse effects than most other anticonvulsants.
- Patients should be given an information leaflet describing how to recognize haematological and hepatic adverse effects of sodium valproate.
- Sodium valproate is teratogenic and is associated with congenital abnormalities, including spina bifida. Counselling and antenatal screening are recommended, as well as regular folate for pregnant women on sodium valproate.

SUMATRIPTAN

Class: Serotonin (5-HT$_1$) agonist

Indications
* Acute migraine.
* Cluster headache (SC use only).

Mechanism of action
* Sumatriptan selectively stimulates the inhibitory serotonin (5-HT$_1$) receptors in the raphe nucleus of the brain. It thereby maintains vasoconstrictor tone, mainly in the carotid arterial circulation. This action is believed to reduce the severity of acute migraine attacks.

Adverse effects
* *Common*: pain at the injection site, flushing, tingling sensation.
* *Rare*: chest tightness or pain, dizziness, lethargy.

Contraindications
* Ischaemic heart disease (sumatriptan produces a small degree of vasoconstriction in coronary vessels).
* Peripheral vascular disease, previous stroke, TIAs, Prinzmetal's angina.
* Severe hypertension.

Interactions
* *Ergotamine*: concomitant use of ergotamine and sumatriptan increases the risk of coronary vasospasm.
* *Lithium*: concomitant use of lithium and sumatriptan increases the risk of CNS toxicity.
* *MAOIs*: concomitant use of MAOIs and sumatriptan increases the risk of CNS toxicity.
* *SSRIs*: concomitant use of SSRIs and sumatriptan increases the risk of CNS toxicity.

Route of administration
* Oral, intranasal spray, SC.

Note
* In acute migraine, simple analgesics such as paracetamol or NSAIDs should be tried first. If these are ineffective, triptans can be used.
* Sumatriptan should be given as soon as possible after the onset of a migraine attack.
* It is more effective if given SC due to poor oral bioavailability and because gastric emptying and absorption is reduced during a migraine attack.

Related drugs
* Almotriptan, eletriptan, frovatriptan, naratriptan, rizatriptan, zolmitriptan.

PSYCHIATRY

Management guidelines

DEPRESSION
• Medical treatment is not usually required for mild depression.
Instead consider:
  • Regular review, psychological interventions (problem-solving therapy, CBT and counselling), exercise, management of sleep and anxiety.
• Only start antidepressants if the above fail, or there is a history of depression.
• First-line drug therapy: SSRI (e.g. fluoxetine).
• If still symptomatic, consider another antidepressant, combination therapy and augmentation with lithium.
• Second-line drugs: another SSRI, lofepramine, mirtazapine, moclobemide, reboxetine, another TCA, venlafaxine.
• Improvement is not usually seen until 2–6 weeks after starting treatment.

The Hands–on Guide to Clinical Pharmacology, 3rd Edition. By S Chatu.
Published 2010 by Blackwell Publishing Ltd.

- For a rapid response and for patients not responding to antidepressants consider electroconvulsive therapy (ECT).
- Inpatient treatment should be considered for those with depression that are at risk of suicide or self harm.
- For those with psychotic symptoms, consider adjunctive treatment with antipsychotic medication.
- Psychotherapy and counselling are of benefit to some patients. CBT is equally as effective as pharmacological treatment.

BIPOLAR DISORDER
- For prophylactic treatment, consider lithium or sodium valproate or olanzapine as monotherapy.
- However, if having frequent relapse or poor control, switch to an alternative from these drugs or consider the use of either two in combination.
- Consider psychological therapy, e.g. CBT.
- If still symptomatic, refer to specialist centre for consideration of ECT, lamotrigine, carbamazepine, antipsychotics and antidepressants.
- Seek specialist advice to treat acute manic and depressive episodes.

DEMENTIA
- Exclude reversible causes of dementia, e.g. normal pressure hydrocephalus, vitamin B_{12} deficiency.
- In Alzheimer's disease, consider acetylcholinesterase inhibitors (donepezil, galantamine or rivastigmine) if Mini Mental State Examination (MMSE) is 10–20 points out of 30.
- Review MMSE and the patient's functional, global and behavioural state every 6 months and only continue with medication if MMSE at, or above, 10 and appropriate to do so.
- To obtain behavioural control in the acute setting, use IM haloperidol, lorazepam or olanzapine.
- Often antipsychotic drugs are used to control behavioural problems and/or psychotic symptoms that can occur with dementia; risperidone and olanzapine increase risk of stroke in the elderly, hence not recommended.
- Depression is a common problem that can be associated with dementia and is managed with antidepressants.

SCHIZOPHRENIA
- Offer CBT to all those with schizophrenia.
- Family intervention therapy should be considered for those in close contact with the patient, to help cope with the illness.
- Offer oral antipsychotic drugs to patients with newly diagnosed schizophrenia (atypical neuroleptics are the preferred choice as they are better tolerated).
- IM depot preparations of antipsychotic medication should be considered in those who are non-compliant.
- ECT may be considered for catatonic schizophrenia.

Drugs types

ANTIDEPRESSANTS
Types
1. *TCAs*:
   - Sedating: amitriptyline, clomipramine, dosulepin, doxepin, trimipramine.
   - Less sedating: imipramine, lofepramine, nortriptyline.
2. *TCA-related antidepressants*: mianserin, trazodone.
3. *SSRIs*: citalopram, escitalopram, fluoxetine, fluvoxamine, paroxetine, sertraline
4. *MAOIs*:
   - Irreversible inhibitors: isocarboxazid, phenelzine, tranylcypromine (these have alerting rather than sedating properties).
   - Reversible inhibitors: moclobemide.
5. *Others*: duloxetine, mirtazapine, reboxetine, tryptophan, venlafaxine.

Note
- SSRIs are better tolerated and safer in overdose than other antidepressants and should be used first line in the treatment of depression.
- Cardiotoxic and antimuscarinic adverse effects in overdose make TCAs undesirable for use in patients at risk of taking overdoses (lofepramine is the only TCA that is relatively safe in overdose).
- SSRIs are less sedating than TCAs and have fewer cardiotoxic and antimuscarinic effects.
- Antidepressants should be withdrawn gradually. Sudden withdrawal may precipitate withdrawal symptoms.
- MAOIs are second-line agents after TCAs and SSRIs due to their hazardous drug and food interactions.
- SSRIs are also used in the treatment of generalized anxiety disorder, obsessive compulsive disorder and panic attacks.

BENZODIAZEPINES
Types
1. *Short-acting*: chlordiazepoxide, loprazolam, lorazepam, lormetazepam, midazolam, temazepam.
2. *Long-acting*: alprazolam, clobazam, clonazepam, diazepam, flurazepam, nitrazepam, oxazepam.

Indications
- Anxiety states (diazepam).
- Insomnia (flurazepam, nitrazepam, temazepam).
- Convulsions (lorazepam or diazepam in status epilepticus, clonazepam and clobazam for prophylaxis).
- Sedation for medical procedures (midazolam).
- Alcohol withdrawal (chlordiazepoxide, diazepam).

Mechanism of action
* Benzodiazepines potentiate the inhibitory actions of GABA by binding to GABA receptors in the CNS.

Adverse effects
* These are usually due to CNS effects: sedation, memory disturbance, blurred vision, ataxia, dysarthria, incontinence, nightmares, confusion, excessive salivation, respiratory depression.
* If used for more than several weeks, benzodiazepines can lead to tolerance and psychological/physical dependence (especially short-acting benzodiazepines). Therefore, treatment should not exceed 2 weeks at a time.

Withdrawing benzodiazepines after long-term treatment
* Arrange a 'contract' with the patient in order to increase compliance.
* In order to avoid withdrawal symptoms, reduce the dose by one-eighth every 2–4 weeks.
* Abrupt withdrawal of benzodiazepines can cause anxiety, tremor, seizures and rebound sleeplessness.

NEUROLEPTICS/ANTIPSYCHOTIC DRUGS
Types
1. Typical:
   * *Phenothiazines*: chlorpromazine, fluphenazine, levomepromazine, pericyazine, perphenazine, pipothiazine, prochlorperazine, promazine, trifluoperazine.
   * *Butyrophenones*: benperidol, haloperidol.
   * *Thioxanthenes*: flupentixol, zuclopenthixol.
   * *Others*: pimozide, sulpiride.
2. Atypical:
   * Amisulpride, aripiprazole, clozapine, olanzapine, paliperidone, quetiapine, risperidone, zotepine.

Indications
* Psychotic symptoms associated with dementia, acute delirium, depression, drug-induced, acute mania.
* In schizophrenia:
  * Typicals are effective for positive symptoms.
  * Atypicals are effective for both negative and positive symptoms.

Mechanism of action
* Exact mechanism is not fully understood.
* All neuroleptics block D_2 receptors in the brain. This is thought to be responsible for the antipsychotic effect.
* Atypicals additionally block $5-HT_2$ receptors in the CNS.

Adverse effects
* D_2-receptor blockade: parkinsonism, depression, hyperprolactinaemia, tardive dyskinesia.
* Muscarinic-receptor blockade: dry mouth, blurred vision, constipation.

- Alpha$_1$-adrenoceptor blockade: postural hypotension.
- H$_1$-receptor blockade: sedation.
- A rare but serious adverse effect is neuroleptic malignant syndrome.
- Atypical neuroleptics may cause weight gain, diabetes and tiredness; they cause less extrapyramidal side-effects.

Note
- Clozapine is used in the treatment of schizophrenia when other antipsychotics are ineffective or not tolerated but is associated with a risk of agranulocytosis and regular blood monitoring is required.
- Atypicals may be better tolerated than typical neuroleptics.
- Risperidone and olanzapine are associated with an increased risk of stroke in elderly patients with dementia.

Drugs

ACETYLCHOLINESTERASE INHIBITORS

(Donepezil, galantamine, rivastigmine)

Indications
* Alzheimer's disease if MMSE 10–20 points.

Mechanism of action
* These drugs increase levels of acetylcholine in the brain by acting as reversible inhibitors of the enzyme acetylcholinesterase thus preventing hydrolysis of acetylcholine. Increased levels of acetylcholine are thought to improve symptoms of dementia such as cognition and behaviour but do not slow down disease progression.

Adverse effects
* *Common*: nausea, vomiting.
* *Rare*: peptic ulcers, GI tract bleeding, seizures, bradyarrhythmias, extrapyramidal symptoms.

Contraindications
* Nil.

Interactions
* *Erythromycin, paroxetine*: these drugs increase the plasma concentration of galantamine.

Route of administration
* Oral.

Note
* Rivastigmine can also be used in dementia associated with Parkinson's disease.
* Regular review is required and treatment should be stopped if MMSE is below 10 or patient not responding.

AMITRIPTYLINE

Class: Tricyclic antidepressant (TCA)

Indications
* Depression.
* Neuropathic pain, e.g. peripheral neuropathy, carpel tunnel syndrome.

Mechanism of action
* Amitriptyline increases serotonin and norepinephrine transmission in the CNS by inhibiting their re-uptake at the synaptic cleft.
* Amitriptyline also blocks H_1-, muscarinic- and alpha$_1$ receptors, which can result in a wide range of adverse effects.

Adverse effects
* *Common*: sedation, dry mouth, blurred vision, postural hypotension, constipation.
* *Rare*: convulsions, cardiac dysrhythmias, weight gain, difficulty in passing urine, precipitation of glaucoma, hyponatraemia, hepatic impairment.

Contraindications
* Recent MI.
* Cardiac dysrhythmias (especially heart block).

Interactions
* *Antiarrhythmics*: amitriptyline increases the risk of ventricular dysrhythmias if given with antiarrhythmics.
* *Anticonvulsants*: amitriptyline antagonises the anticonvulsant effect.
* *MAOIs*: danger of potentially fatal hyperthermia syndrome.
* *Neuroleptics*: increased risk of ventricular dysrhythmias.

Route of administration
* Oral.

Note
* Amitriptyline must be taken regularly for 3–4 weeks before any improvement is likely.
* Used in the treatment of irritable bowel syndrome when antispasmodics, laxatives and antidiarrhoeal agents are ineffective.
* Amitriptyline is not recommended in the treatment of depression as it is dangerous in overdose; other TCAs are preferred and used as second line agents if SSRIs are ineffective or not tolerated.
* Amitriptyline can be used for the prophylactic treatment of migraine.

Related drugs
* Sedating: clomipramine, dosulepin, doxepin, trimipramine.
* Non-sedating: imipramine, lofepramine, nortriptyline.

CHLORPROMAZINE

Class: Phenothiazine

Indications

* Psychotic disorders (e.g. schizophrenia, mania).
* Labyrinthine disturbances and vertigo.
* Nausea and vomiting.
* Chronic hiccups.

Mechanism of action

* Exact mechanism is not fully understood.
* In psychotic disorders chlorpromazine is thought to block D_2 receptors in the CNS, especially in the mesocortical and mesolimbic areas.
* The antiemetic effect is due to blockade of D_2 receptors in the chemoreceptor trigger zone in the brain.
* Blockade of muscarinic-, H_1-, serotonin- and alpha receptors might contribute to the therapeutic action of chlorpromazine, but also causes adverse effects.

Adverse effects

* *Common*: sedation, postural hypotension, raised prolactin levels (leading to subfertility, impotence, menstrual disturbances, galactorrhoea), extrapyramidal adverse effects (acute dystonia, akathisia, parkinsonism, tardive dyskinesia with long-term use), anticholinergic effects (e.g. dry mouth, blurred vision).
* *Rare*: neuroleptic malignant syndrome (hyperthermia, muscle rigidity, autonomic nervous system dysfunction), agranulocytosis, photosensitive rash, jaundice.

Contraindications

* Coma.
* Bone marrow suppression.
* Phaeochromocytoma.
* Pregnancy and breastfeeding.

Interactions

* *ACE inhibitors*: these can cause severe postural hypotension if given with chlorpromazine.

Route of administration

* Oral, rectal, IM.

Note

* Compliance may be a problem in psychotic patients. In this case slow-release preparations of other neuroleptics (e.g. haloperidol decanoate) can be given IM every few weeks.
* Extrapyramidal adverse effects are thought to be due to the blockade of dopamine receptors in the CNS.
* Chlorpromazine can be used in conjunction with an anticholinergic drug (e.g. procyclidine) to prevent short-term extrapyramidal adverse effects. However, this cannot prevent tardive dyskinesia.

Related drugs

* Fluphenazine, levomepromazine, pericyazine, perphenazine, pipothiazine, prochlorperazine, trifluoperazine.

HALOPERIDOL

Class: Butyrophenone D_2 antagonist

Indications
- Schizophrenia and other psychotic disorders.
- Motor tics.
- Short-term sedation of acutely violent or otherwise agitated patients (e.g. in dementia).
- Nausea and vomiting in terminally ill patients.

Mechanism of action
- Haloperidol blocks postsynaptic D_2 receptors in the limbic, striatal and cortical brain regions.
- It also blocks D_1 receptors, but to a much lesser extent.

Adverse effects
- *Common*: extrapyramidal effects with long-term use (e.g. parkinsonism, acute dystonia, akathisia), drowsiness, postural hypotension.
- *Rare*: weight loss, tardive dyskinesia, convulsions, neuroleptic malignant syndrome, jaundice, blood dyscrasias.

Contraindications
- Coma.
- Bone marrow suppression.

Interactions
- *Amiodarone*: haloperidol increases risk of ventricular dysrhythmias.
- *Carbamazepine*: decreases the plasma concentration of haloperidol by accelerating its metabolism.
- *Fluoxetine*: increases the plasma concentration of haloperidol.

Route of administration
- Oral, IM.

Note
- Haloperidol requires several weeks to exert control over the symptoms of schizophrenia.
- Extrapyramidal adverse effects (e.g. parkinsonism, akathisia) can be ameliorated by giving muscarinic antagonists (e.g. procyclidine) or by reducing the dose.
- In order to avoid first-pass metabolism and improve compliance, haloperidol can be given every 1–4 weeks as a long-acting, deep depot IM injection (given as haloperidol decanoate).
- Haloperidol, as well as any other neuroleptic agent, can cause the potentially fatal neuroleptic malignant syndrome (hyperpyrexia, confusion, increased muscle tone and autonomic dysfunction). There is no effective treatment for this, apart from immediate discontinuation of the causative drug. In some cases it may be treated with dantrolene or bromocriptine.
- Haloperidol is often used to obtain behavioural control in patients with acute delirium or dementia in hospitalized patients.

Related drugs
- Benperidol, droperidol.

LITHIUM

Class: Mood stabilizer

Indications
* Treatment and prophylaxis of mania.
* Prophylaxis of bipolar affective disorder.
* Resistant recurrent depression.

Mechanism of action
* Exact mechanism is not fully understood.
* Lithium is thought to:
   1. Reduce glutamatergic activity in the CNS.
   2. Act upon signal mechanisms in the CNS (adenylyl cyclase, glycogen synthase kinase-3 beta, cAMP).
   3. Inhibit second messengers in the CNS.
* All of these actions are believed to assist in stabilizing neuronal activity.

Adverse effects
* *Common*: weight gain, nausea, vomiting, diarrhoea, tremor.
* *Rare*: renal tubular damage (nephrogenic diabetes insipidus, interstitial nephritis), hypothyroidism, muscle weakness, drowsiness, blurred vision, rash, memory impairment (in long-term use), cardiac dysrhythmias, hyperthyroidism.

Contraindications
* None.
* Caution:
   * Renal impairment (lithium is excreted renally).
   * Cardiac disease.
   * Pregnancy and breastfeeding.
   * Elderly.

Interactions
* *Diuretics*: increase the plasma concentration of lithium by reducing its excretion.
* *SSRIs*: increase the risk of lithium adverse effects.

Route of administration
* Oral.

Note
* An ECG should be taken prior to starting lithium (risk of cardiac dysrhythmias).
* Thyroid and renal function must be tested prior to and during treatment with lithium because of its potential nephrotoxic and thyrotoxic effects.
* Lithium has a narrow therapeutic window. Plasma concentration must therefore be monitored, as overdose can be fatal.
* Lithium toxicity manifests as drowsiness, confusion, ataxia, seizures and coma. Management of toxicity includes increasing fluid intake and providing supportive treatment. Haemodialysis can be performed in severe cases.
* Sodium competes with lithium for re-absorption in the renal tubules. Therefore, hyponatraemia can increase the risk of lithium toxicity.

MIRTAZAPINE

Class: Antidepressant

Indications
* Depression.

Mechanism of action
* Enhances noradrenaline and serotonin transmission in the CNS.

Adverse effects
* *Common*: weight gain, sedation, tiredness.
* *Rare*: dizziness, postural hypotension, rash, blood disorders, seizures, lucid dreams.

Contraindications
* Nil.

Interactions
* *Warfarin*: anticoagulant effect is enhanced by mirtazapine.
* *MAOIs*: mirtazapine should not be started until 2 weeks after stopping MAOIs and vice versa.
* *Carbamazepine, phenytoin*: these reduce the plasma concentration of mirtazapine.
* *Sibutramine*: increased risk of CNS toxicity if used in conjunction with mirtazapine.

Route of administration
* Oral.

Note
* If treatment is to be stopped then the dose should be reduced gradually over a few weeks to prevent withdrawal syndrome (nausea, vomiting, anxiety, dizziness, headache).
* If the patient develops signs of an infection, an urgent FBC should be checked and the drug stopped if there is evidence of neutropenia.
* Mirtazapine is relatively safe in overdose.
* Mirtazapine tends to cause sedation at lower doses due to its antihistamine effects. However, at higher doses it has a stimulatory effect due to its adrenergic effect overpowering the antihistamine effect.

PHENELZINE

Class: Monoamine oxidase inhibitor (MAOI)

Indications
* Depression.

Mechanism of action
* Causes non-selective irreversible inhibition of the enzyme MAO type A involved in the metabolism of serotonin, norepinephrine and dopamine. Consequently, their concentrations are increased in the brain, peripheral neurons, gut wall and platelets.
* MAO in the gut wall normally metabolizes tyramine in foodstuffs. If tyramine-containing food is ingested while on phenelzine, this can lead to an accumulation of tyramine, which in turn causes a rise in norepinephrine levels. This can trigger a hypertensive crisis.

Adverse effects
* *Common*: dizziness, blurred vision, postural hypotension, dry mouth.
* *Rare*: hypertensive crisis, hepatotoxicity, rash, drowsiness, constipation.

Contraindications
* Hepatic impairment.
* Cerebrovascular disease.
* Phaeochromocytoma.

Interactions
* *Levodopa and sympathomimetics*: increased risk of a hypertensive crisis (sweating, restlessness, flushing, hyperpyrexia, tremor, convulsions, coma).
* *SSRIs, TCAs*: predisposition to CNS excitation and hypertension.
* *Tyramine-containing foods* (e.g. pickled herring, cheese, wine, beer, yeast, chocolate): risk of a hypertensive crisis.

Route of administration
* Oral.

Note
* Owing to its drug and food interactions (especially with tyramine-rich foods) phenelzine is usually a third- line drug for the treatment of depression after TCAs and SSRIs.
* MAOIs should not be started until at least 2 weeks after a previous MAOI, TCA or SSRI has been stopped (5 weeks for fluoxetine, owing to longer half-life).
* Other antidepressants should not be started for 2 weeks after treatment with an MAOI has been stopped.
* Patients should carry a warning card, detailing which foods should be avoided (see above under Interactions).
* Phenelzine is metabolized by acetylation. Slow acetylators (about half the population of Europe and the USA) are more likely to develop adverse effects.

Related drugs
* Isocarboxazid, tranylcypromine.

RISPERIDONE

Class: Benzisoxazole derivative ('atypical' neuroleptic)

Indications
• Psychosis (acute or chronic).

Mechanism of action
• Exact mechanism is not fully understood.
• Atypical neuroleptics are believed to achieve their effect by blocking D_2- and 5-HT_2 receptors in the brain.

Adverse effects
• *Common*: weight gain, headache, anxiety, insomnia, postural hypotension, dizziness.
• *Rare*: constipation, tardive dyskinesia, neuroleptic malignant syndrome, blurred vision, cardiac dysrhythmias, hyperprolactinaemia, hyperglycaemia, seizures.

Contraindications
• Breastfeeding.

Interactions
• *Antihypertensives*: enhanced hypotensive effect with atypical neuroleptics.
• *Avoid drugs that prolong the QT interval with amisulpride.*
• *Avoid drugs that have the potential to cause agranulocytosis with clozapine.*
• Many other interactions exist.

Route of administration
• Oral.

Note
• Risperidone is especially useful for controlling 'negative' as well as 'positive' symptoms in schizophrenia.
• Before starting treatment with atypical neuroleptics an ECG should be taken to assess the QT interval.
• Clozapine is used in the treatment of schizophrenia and requires regular monitoring of the full blood count as it may cause agranulocytosis.
• Quetiapine is often used first line to control behavioural problems in elderly patients with dementia.
• Risperidone and olanzapine increase the risk of stroke in elderly patients with dementia so should be avoided in this group.

Related drugs
• Other 'atypical' neuroleptics: amisulpride, aripiprazole, clozapine, olanzapine, quetiapine, zotepine.

SELECTIVE SEROTONIN RE-UPTAKE INHIBITORS (SSRIs)

(Citalopram, escitalopram, fluoxetine, fluvoxamine, paroxetine, sertraline)

Class: SSRIs

Indications
* Depression.
* Obsessive–compulsive disorder.
* Generalized anxiety disorder.
* Panic attacks.

Mechanism of action
* SSRIs increase serotonin levels in the CNS by inhibiting its re-uptake from the synaptic cleft.

Adverse effects
* *Common*: headache, insomnia, nausea, abdominal pain, diarrhoea, anxiety, sexual dysfunction.
* *Rare*: anaphylaxis, drowsiness, serotonin syndrome (agitation, confusion, fever, trembling), constipation.

Contraindications
* Mania.

Interactions
* *Carbamazepine*: fluoxetine increases the plasma concentration of carbamazepine.
* *Dopaminergics*: fluoxetine causes hypertension and CNS excitation if given with dopaminergics.
* *Lithium*: fluoxetine increases the risk of lithium toxicity.
* *Phenytoin*: fluoxetine increases the plasma concentration of phenytoin.

Route of administration
* Oral.

Note
* SSRIs are preferred to TCAs because they are safer in overdose. SSRIs are relatively free of anticholinergic adverse effects, such as blurred vision, dry mouth and difficult micturition. SSRIs are less sedating and cardiotoxic than TCAs.
* After stopping fluoxetine, active substances may persist in the body for weeks. This must be borne in mind when prescribing new drugs with the potential to interact with fluoxetine.
* SSRIs should not be started until 14 days after stopping an MAOI.
* SSRIs increase the risk of GI bleeding if used in conjunction with aspirin.
* SSRIs may increase the risk of suicide and self harm in children and adolescents (except for fluoxetine), hence careful monitoring is required.

TEMAZEPAM

Class: Benzodiazepine

Indications
- Insomnia.
- Premedication before surgery.

Mechanism of action
- Temazepam binds to GABA receptors in the CNS and thereby facilitates GABA-inhibitory neurotransmission by opening chloride channels. This action is thought to produce the sedative and anxiolytic effects.

Adverse effects
- *Common*: drowsiness and light headedness next day, confusion and ataxia in the elderly.
- *Rare*: amnesia.

Contraindications
- Respiratory depression (may be worsened by temazepam).
- Severe hepatic impairment.
- Myasthenia gravis.
- Sleep apnoea syndrome.

Interactions
- *Alcohol*: this enhances the sedative effect of temazepam.

Route of administration
- Oral.

Note
- Temazepam should only be used short term to avoid psychological and physical dependence.
- Flumazenil can be used as an antidote to temazepam overdose.
- Nitrazepam, flurazepam, loprazolam and lormetazepam are benzodiazepines that are used in the short-term treatment of insomnia.
- Zopiclone is a non-benzodiazepine that can be used as an alternative in the treatment of insomnia.

ZOPICLONE

Class: Cyclopyrrolone hypnotic

Indications
* Insomnia.

Mechanism of action
* Zopiclone acts in a similar way to benzodiazepines but causes less sedation, less dependence and less muscle relaxation.
* It binds to the benzodiazepine receptor complex in the CNS, facilitating the actions of GABA, an inhibitory neurotransmitter.

Adverse effects
* *Common*: bitter taste in the mouth, GI effects (anorexia, abdominal pain, constipation).
* *Rare*: mood changes, dependence (with long-term use), palpitations, agitation, trembling.

Contraindications
* Myasthenia gravis.
* Respiratory failure.
* Severe sleep apnoea.
* Severe hepatic impairment.
* Pregnancy and breastfeeding.

Interactions
* *Erythromycin*: this inhibits the metabolism of zopiclone.

Route of administration
* Oral.

Note
* Non-drug therapy should be tried prior to starting zopiclone.
* Zopiclone lengthens the duration of sleep and reduces the number of nocturnal awakenings.
* Overdose manifests as confusion, ataxia and drowsiness. This should be managed with gastric lavage, IV fluids and observation.
* Continuous treatment with zopiclone should not exceed 2–4 weeks. Continued use may result in dependence.
* Zopiclone causes less 'morning-after' drowsiness than long-acting benzodiazepines.

Related drugs
* Zaleplon, zolpidem.

MUSCULOSKELETAL SYSTEM

Management guidelines (pp. 111–113)
Gout
Osteoarthritis
Osteoporosis
Rheumatoid arthritis

Drug types (p. 114)
Corticosteroids

Drugs (pp. 115–124)
Allopurinol
Azathioprine
Biologics/cytokine modulators
Bisphosphonates
Calcitonin
Cyclo-oxygenase-2 (COX-2) inhibitors
Cyclophosphamide
Methotrexate
Penicillamine
Prednisolone

Management guidelines

GOUT
Acute gout
- In an acute attack give NSAIDs (e.g. indomethacin) but *not* aspirin, as it inhibits uric acid excretion.
- If NSAIDs are contraindicated, give colchicine or corticosteroids.

Prevention
- Regular treatment to reduce uric acid levels is required for frequent recurrent attacks of gout, or if gouty tophi present, or if chronic arthritis due to gout.
- Reduce intake of excessive alcohol and purine-rich foods (oily fish, liver, kidney).
- Encourage weight loss if appropriate.
- Consider allopurinol to decrease uric acid synthesis, or a uricosuric drug (i.e. probenecid, sulfinpyrazone and benzbromarone) to increase urinary uric acid excretion.

The Hands–on Guide to Clinical Pharmacology, 3rd Edition. By S Chatu.
Published 2010 by Blackwell Publishing Ltd.

- Usually start preventative medication with colchicine or NSAID to prevent an acute attack and continue until at least hyperuricaemia has been corrected.

OSTEOARTHRITIS
- Recommend regular physical exercise to maintain muscle bulk and joint mobility.
- Reduce weight if appropriate.
- Supply walking aid if necessary.
- Paracetamol, local NSAID gels and systemic NSAIDs for pain control.
- Intra-articular steroid injections are useful for inflammatory exacerbations.
- Other options for pain control are glucosamine for osteoarthritis of the knee, topical capsaicin gel and in severe pain opiates may be required.
- Consider joint replacement if pain and loss of joint function are not improved by analgesics and exercise.

OSTEOPOROSIS
Prevention
- Advise lifestyle measures, such as regular exercise, cessation of smoking, avoiding excess alcohol and avoiding immobility.
- Maintain adequate calcium and vitamin D intake. Give supplements if necessary.
- In the frail elderly, consider hip-protector pants to prevent fractures from falls.

Treatment
- Confirm osteoporosis with bone densitometry (except in patients aged 75 years and over who should routinely be given osteoporosis treatment after any fracture as a preventative measure).
- If between 65 and 74 years old, treat if T-score is below -2.5 on dual energy X-ray absorptiometry (DEXA) scan.
- If under 65 years, treat if T-score is -3 or below with other risk factors, i.e. body mass index (BMI) <19; two or more vertebral fractures; maternal hip fracture under 75 years old; early menopause; conditions associated with prolonged immobility; chronic medical conditions associated with increased risk of osteoporosis, e.g. rheumatoid arthritis, inflammatory bowel disease.
- Advise lifestyle changes (as per prevention).
- Maintain adequate calcium and vitamin D intake. Give supplements if necessary.
- Give a bisphosphonate (e.g. alendronic acid) or strontium ranelate if bisphosphonate is contraindicated, intolerable or ineffective.
- If bisphosphonate and strontium ranelate are inappropriate, consider these alternatives:
    - Raloxifene (selective oestrogen-receptor modulator).
    - Teriparatide, a parathyroid hormone (PTH) analogue.
    - Intranasal calcitonin.
    - Hormone replacement therapy (HRT).

RHEUMATOID ARTHRITIS

* Multidisciplinary team approach is important (education, physiotherapy, joint protection, walking aids, orthotics, social services, general practitioner [GP] and specialist).
* Recommend regular physical exercise to maintain muscle bulk and joint mobility.

Medical treatment

* First-line therapy:
    * Disease-modifying antirheumatic drugs (methotrexate and sometimes sulfasalazine) slow disease progression and alter inflammatory markers but require monitoring.
    * Paracetamol and NSAIDs for symptomatic relief (e.g. ibuprofen, celecoxib).
* Second-line therapy: alternative disease-modifying antirheumatic drug (DMARDs) (i.e. leflunomide, penicillamine, gold, hydroxychloroquine, azathioprine). Penicillamine and gold are not commonly used now.
* Recent evidence shows that a combination of DMARDs with or without corticosteroids early in the course of disease is associated with a better outcome.
* Anti-TNF antibodies (i.e. infliximab, etanercept) can be used for active disease not responding to two or more conventional DMARDs.
* Rituximab, a monoclonal antibody against CD20 B cells, is also licensed for rheumatoid arthritis.
* Corticosteroids can be given for an anti-inflammatory effect:
    * Orally.
    * Parenterally – IM long-acting depot injection or large bolus given IV.
    * Locally – injection into an inflamed joint.

Surgical treatment

* Surgery is an option for some patients (e.g. carpal tunnel decompression, synovectomy, tendon repair, arthrodesis, arthroplasty).

Drug types

CORTICOSTEROIDS

Types of corticosteroids

1. *Glucocorticoids*: beclomethasone, cortisone, dexamethasone, hydrocortisone, methylprednisolone, prednisolone, triamcinolone.

2. *Mineralocorticoids*: fludrocortisone.

Indications

- *Glucocorticoids* are mainly used for:
  - Suppression of inflammation.
  - Suppression of the immune system.
  - Replacement therapy, e.g. Addison's disease.
  - Part of chemotherapy (in Hodgkin's lymphoma and acute leukaemia).
  - Reduction of oedema (e.g. in brain tumours).
- *Mineralocorticoids* are mainly used in replacement therapy and treatment of postural hypotension.

Adverse effects

- Glucocorticoid effects: cushingoid appearance, osteoporosis, growth suppression, diabetes mellitus, peptic ulcer, cataract, glaucoma, susceptibility to infection, impaired wound healing, easy bruising.
- Mineralocorticoid effects: hypokalaemia and hypertension (secondary to sodium and water retention).
- Note: topical use of corticosteroids limits systemic adverse effects.

Drugs

ALLOPURINOL

Class: Antigout agent

Indications
- Prophylaxis of gout.
- Prophylaxis of uric acid and calcium oxalate renal stones.
- Prophylaxis of hyperuricaemia secondary to chemotherapy.

Mechanism of action
- Allopurinol decreases uric acid production by inhibiting the enzyme xanthine oxidase, which converts xanthine to uric acid. The excess xanthine is easily excreted as it is more soluble.

Adverse effects
- *Common*: rash.
- *Rare*: headache, seizures, metallic taste in the mouth, blood disorders, Stevens–Johnson syndrome, hypersensitivity reactions, hepatotoxicity.

Contraindications
- Acute gout attack.
- Caution:
    - Renal impairment (allopurinol is renally excreted).

Interactions
- *Ampicillin, amoxicillin*: increased risk of a rash.
- *Azathioprine, mercaptopurine*: the effects of these drugs are enhanced by allopurinol.
- *Ciclosporin, warfarin*: allopurinol may enhance the effect of these drugs.

Route of administration
- Oral.

Note
- The risk of a gout attack is increased in the first few weeks of treatment with allopurinol. This can be avoided by taking allopurinol with an NSAID (not aspirin) or colchicine until hyperuricaemia is corrected.
- High fluid intake during allopurinol therapy is recommended (approximately 2 L/day).
- Rasburicase is another drug that can be used for preventing and treating acute hyperuricaemia during chemotherapy and is used in haematological malignancies.

AZATHIOPRINE

Class: Immunosuppressive agent

Indications
- Autoimmune diseases (e.g. rheumatoid arthritis, SLE).
- Prevention of transplant rejection.
- Used as a steroid-sparing drug (in severe inflammatory conditions e.g. Crohn's disease, ulcerative colitis).

Mechanism of action
- Azathioprine is metabolized to 6-mercaptopurine in the liver. This metabolite is taken up into cells, where it inhibits DNA synthesis by interfering with purine metabolism. Azathioprine thus has a cytotoxic effect on dividing cells.
- Azathioprine also has an immunosuppressive effect on cells.

Adverse effects
- *Common*: nausea, vomiting, bone marrow suppression.
- *Rare*: alopecia, arthralgia, liver impairment, pancreatitis, renal impairment.

Contraindications
- Hypersensitivity.

Interactions
- *Allopurinol*: inhibits the metabolism of azathioprine, thus increasing the risk of adverse effects.
- *Antibacterials*: rifampicin, co-trimoxazole and trimethoprim enhance the risk of toxicity with azathioprine.
- *Warfarin*: effect of warfarin possibly reduced.

Route of administration
- Oral, IV (very irritant and only rarely used).

Note
- Azathioprine is potentially highly toxic. Close monitoring is required, whereby FBC, LFTs and renal function are checked regularly (at least 2-3 monthly) to detect bone marrow suppression, liver or renal impairment.
- Bone marrow suppression may manifest as bleeding, bruising, fatigue or repeated infections.
- Thiopurine methyltransferase (TPMT) levels are usually checked before treatment is commenced. This enzyme metabolizes azathioprine and its deficiency increases the risk of bone marrow suppression with azathioprine.
- Azathioprine is used in the treatment of IBD in those who are dependant or resistant to steroids.

BIOLOGICS/CYTOKINE MODULATORS

(Infliximab, adalimumab, etanercept, rituximab)

Indications
- Rheumatological conditions: rheumatoid arthritis, psoriatic arthritis, ankylosing spondylitis.
- Inflammatory bowel disease.
- Psoriasis.

Mechanism of action
- Tumour necrosis factor (TNF) alpha induces inflammatory cytokines and hence its suppression has an anti-inflammatory effect.
- Infliximab and adalimumab are monoclonal antibodies that inhibit TNF alpha activity.
- Etanercept is a TNF receptor, which neutralizes the circulating TNF.
- Rituximab is a monoclonal antibody against CD20B cells.

Adverse effects
- *Common*: infections, local injection reactions, GI side-effects, worsening of heart failure.
- *Rare*: lupus-like disease, blood disorders (anaemia, leucopenia, thrombocytopenia, aplastic anaemia), demyelinating CNS disease.

Contraindications
- Pregnancy and breastfeeding.
- Severe infections.

Interactions
- *Live vaccines*: avoid live vaccines while receiving cytokine modulators.

Route of administration
- SC, IV.

Note
- Rituximab originally approved for the treatment of lymphoma can now be used in rheumatoid arthritis (in conjunction with methotrexate) if anti-TNF therapy fails.
- Careful screening for chronic infections (e.g. tuberculosis) and malignancy is important before the initiation of treatment.
- All three anti-TNF drugs are licensed for the treatment of rheumatoid arthritis, psoriatic arthritis and ankylosing spondylitis.
- Biologics are not recommended in those with moderate to severe cardiac failure or demyelinating disorders because symptoms may worsen.

BISPHOSPHONATES

(Alendronic acid, risedronate)

Indications
- Prevention and treatment of osteoporosis.
- Hypercalcaemia of malignancy.
- Metastatic bone malignancy to prevent fractures and reduce pain.
- Paget's disease of the bone.

Mechanism of action
- These drugs inhibit osteoclast activity and hence reduce bone turnover. They improve bone mineralization and increase bone mass.
- Bisphosphonates are thought to achieve their effects through inhibition of a rate-limiting step in cholesterol synthesis, which is essential for the normal function of osteoclasts.

Adverse effects
- *Common*: abdominal discomfort, flatulence, headache.
- *Rare*: oesophageal reactions (oesophageal strictures, ulcers, erosions), peptic ulceration, hypocalcaemia, osteonecrosis of the jaw.

Contraindications
- Oesophageal abnormalities (e.g. achalasia, stricture).
- Pregnancy and breastfeeding.
- Hypocalcaemia.

Interactions
- *Aminoglycosides*: increase the risk of hypocalcaemia.
- *Oral iron, antacids, calcium salts*: reduce absorption of bisphosphonates.

Route of administration
- Oral, IV.

Note
- Ibandronic acid can be given 3 monthly and zoledronic acid yearly as an IV infusion for the treatment of osteoporosis when an oral bisphosphonate is inappropriate.
- Alendronic acid and risedronate are common first-line choices.
- IV pamidronate or zoledronic acid are commonly used to treat hypercalcaemia of malignancy but normalization of calcium can take several days.
- Oesophageal reactions can be prevented by taking oral bisphosphonates with water and remaining seated upright for at least 30 minutes.
- Dental work should be carried out before commencing bisphosphonates as they can rarely cause osteonecrosis of the jaw.

Related drugs
- Disodium etidronate, disodium pamidronate, ibandronic acid, sodium clodronate, tiludronic acid, zoledronic acid.

CALCITONIN

Class: Hormone

Indications
* Paget's disease of bone.
* Hypercalcaemia.
* Bone pain in malignancy.
* Treatment of osteoporosis (post menopausal and steroid-induced).

Mechanism of action
* Calcitonin lowers serum calcium by two main mechanisms:
   1. It decreases bone resorption by inhibiting the activity of osteoclasts and by reducing their number.
   2. It increases renal calcium and phosphate excretion by inhibiting their re-absorption in the tubules.

Adverse effects
* *Common*: nausea, vomiting, flushing.
* *Rare*: tingling in the hand, inflammation at the injection site, unpleasant taste in the mouth.

Contraindications
* Breastfeeding.

Interactions
* None.

Route of administration
* IV, IM, SC, intranasally.

Note
* Two types of calcitonin preparations are available: salmon (natural) and salcatonin (synthetic). Both are immunogenic (antibodies can be made against them), but salcatonin is less so and is thus more suitable in long-term therapy.
* Calcium supplements should be given in conjunction with calcitonin.
* If HRT is not tolerated or is inappropriate, a combination of calcitonin, bisphosphonate and calcium supplements can be used to treat osteoporosis.
* In Paget's disease of bone, calcitonin decreases pain and may prevent neurological complications.

CYCLO-OXYGENASE-2 (COX-2) INHIBITORS

(Celecoxib, etodolac, etoricoxib, meloxicam)

Class: Non-steroidal anti-inflammatory drug (NSAID); COX-2 inhibitor

Indications
- Inflammation and pain in rheumatoid and osteoarthritis.

Mechanism of action
- These drugs inhibit conversion of arachidonic acid into prostaglandin E_2 through selective inhibition of COX-2. This leads to a decrease in:

  1. Vascular permeability and vasodilatation (anti-inflammatory effect).

  2. Sensitization of pain afferents (analgesic effect).

  3. The effect of prostaglandins on the hypothalamus (antipyretic effect).

- COX-1 inhibition is associated with GI adverse effects. Since celecoxib is a specific COX-2 inhibitor, such adverse effects are less (especially when compared to other NSAIDs).

Adverse effects
- *Common*: abdominal discomfort, sinusitis.
- *Rare*: palpitations, GI bleeding, stomatitis, muscle cramps.

Contraindications
- Active peptic ulceration.
- Inflammatory bowel disease.
- Severe heart failure.
- European drug agency recommends not to use COX-2 inhibitors in patients with established atherosclerotic disease, i.e. IHD, stroke, TIA, peripheral vascular disease.

Interactions
- *Fluconazole*: increases plasma concentration of celecoxib.
- *Rifampicin*: reduces concentration of etoricoxib.

Route of administration
- Oral.

Note
- COX-2 inhibitors have a lower risk of upper GI bleeding than non-selective NSAIDs. Other adverse effects are similar to those of non-selective NSAIDs.
- Unlike aspirin, celecoxib has no antiplatelet properties.
- Long-term use of COX-2 inhibitors is thought to increase the risk of thrombotic events (i.e. MI, stroke) and should only be used in preference to NSAIDs after assessing cardiovascular risk and in those at high risk of GI tract ulcers or bleeding.

CYCLOPHOSPHAMIDE

Class: Alkylating agent (immunosuppressive agent)

Indications
- Malignant tumours (lymphomas, chronic lymphocytic leukaemia and solid tumours).
- Vasculitis.
- Autoimmune disease (e.g. SLE).

Mechanism of action
- Cyclophosphamide is inactive until it undergoes hepatic metabolism.
- It damages the deoxyribonucleic acid (DNA) in cells by forming cross-links between strands and by causing base substitution. Consequently, the DNA cannot replicate and this prevents cell division.
- It has an immunosuppressant effect.

Adverse effects
- *Common*: bone marrow suppression, alopecia. High-dose effects: nausea, vomiting, anorexia, change in colour of skin, hair and nails, infertility in men and women.
- *Rare*: haemorrhagic cystitis, cardiotoxic, pulmonary fibrosis.

Contraindications
- Pregnancy and breastfeeding.

Interactions
- *Suxamethonium*: effects of suxamethonium are enhanced by cyclophosphamide.

Route of administration
- Oral, IV.

Note
- While on cyclophosphamide, it is recommended to be taking mesna and to maintain a high fluid intake in order to prevent haemorrhagic cystitis. Mesna neutralizes acrolein, the toxic metabolite of cyclophosphamide, which damages the bladder. Mesna should be continued for about 24–48 hours after stopping cyclophosphamide.
- As cyclophosphamide acts on the testis and ovaries it can increase the risk of infertility. This may be irreversible and a discussion regarding sperm and egg storage should therefore be undertaken with the patient before therapy.
- Long-term use may increase the risk of developing acute myeloid leukaemia and lymphomas.

METHOTREXATE

Class: Immunosuppressive agent

Indications

*   Part of various cancer chemotherapy regimens (e.g. acute lymphoblastic leukaemia, non-Hodgkin's lymphoma, choriocarcinoma).
*   Rheumatoid arthritis.
*   Inflammatory bowel disease.
*   Psoriasis (when conventional therapy has failed).

Mechanism of action

*   Methotrexate is a competitive antagonist of the enzyme dihydrofolate reductase, which catalyses the production of tetrahydrofolic acid from dihydrofolate. This antagonism results in decreased production of tetrahydrofolic acid, which is an essential component for synthesis of nucleic acids (purines and thymidylic acid). Methotrexate therefore inhibits DNA, RNA and protein synthesis, leading to cell death.
*   Methotrexate further suppresses epidermal activity in the skin, hence its use in psoriasis.
*   Mechanism of action in rheumatoid arthritis is not clearly understood.

Adverse effects

*   *Common*: bone marrow suppression, mucositis (e.g. stomatitis, gingivitis), anorexia, nausea, vomiting, diarrhoea, hepatotoxicity (with prolonged treatment).
*   *Rare*: pneumonitis, pulmonary fibrosis, renal impairment.

Contraindications

*   Renal impairment (methotrexate is renally excreted).
*   Hepatic impairment.
*   Pregnancy and breastfeeding.
*   Immunodeficiency syndromes.
*   Active infection.

Interactions

*   *Acitretin*: increases the plasma concentration of methotrexate, thus increasing the risk of hepatotoxicity.
*   *Ciclosporin*: increases methotrexate toxicity.
*   *NSAIDs, probenecid*: increase the risk of methotrexate toxicity by reducing its excretion.

Route of administration

*   Oral, SC, IM, IV, intrathecal.

Note

*   Folinic acid is used to prevent and reverse the toxic effects of methotrexate ('folinic acid rescue') such as mucositis or bone marrow suppression.
*   Methotrexate has teratogenic effects. Contraceptive precautions are therefore necessary during and until 3 months after stopping treatment with methotrexate.
*   Treatment with methotrexate can cause folate deficiency leading to megaloblastic anaemia therefore regular folic acid should also be prescribed.
*   Regular monitoring of FBC, renal and LFTs is recommended, with appropriate dose adjustment or immediate withdrawal of treatment.

PENICILLAMINE

Class: Disease-modifying antirheumatic drug (DMARD)

Indications
- Wilson's disease.
- Copper poisoning.
- Lead poisoning.
- Cystinuria.
- Active rheumatoid arthritis (not commonly used now).

Mechanism of action
- Exact mechanism in rheumatoid arthritis is not fully understood. Penicillamine has immune-modulatory effects by reducing the number of lymphocytes.
- Penicillamine chelates metal ions via its sulphadryl group (hence useful in Wilson's disease and copper/lead poisoning).
- Penicillamine is thought to form a soluble disulphide complex with cystine (hence useful in cystinuria).

Adverse effects
- *Common*: rash, proteinuria, anorexia, nausea, vomiting.
- *Rare*: bone marrow suppression, drug-induced lupus, pemphigus, fever, mouth ulceration, myasthenia gravis, loss of taste.

Contraindications
- Hypersensitivity to penicillin (penicillamine is a degradation product of penicillin).
- SLE.

Interactions
- *Iron*: oral iron reduces the absorption of penicillamine.

Route of administration
- Oral.

Note
- Penicillamine is very rarely used in rheumatoid arthritis nowadays.
- Clinical improvement in rheumatoid arthritis can be expected after 6–12 weeks of treatment. Penicillamine should be stopped if no improvement is evident within 1 year.
- Regular blood and urine tests should be performed to detect any bone marrow suppression or proteinuria.
- Penicillamine should be taken before meals to reduce adverse GI effects.

PREDNISOLONE

Class: Glucocorticoid

Indications
* Anti-inflammatory therapy (e.g. inflammatory bowel disease, asthma, eczema).
* Immunosuppressive therapy (e.g. prevention of transplant rejection, acute leukaemia).
* Glucocorticoid replacement therapy (e.g. Addison's disease).

Mechanism of action
* Prednisolone inhibits phospholipase A_2 activity, which is responsible for the production of free arachidonic acid. Arachidonic acid is the precursor for prostaglandin and leukotriene synthesis. Inhibition of this process therefore achieves an anti-inflammatory effect.
* Prednisolone decreases B and T lymphocyte response to antigens, thus achieving an immunosuppressive effect.

Adverse effects
* *Common*: bruising, hirsutism, moon-face, hypertension, weight gain/oedema, impaired glucose tolerance, acne, cataract, glaucoma, osteoporosis, candida infection, mood changes.
* *Rare*: peptic ulcers, muscle weakness, reactivation of tuberculosis, pancreatitis.

Contraindications
* Systemic infection.

Interactions
* *Ciclosporin*: increases plasma concentration of prednisolone.
* *Phenytoin, carbamazepine*: reduce the effects of prednisolone.

Route of administration
* Oral, IM, IV, topical, rectal.

Note
* Patients on prednisolone should be given a steroid card.
* Prolonged treatment with prednisolone leads to adrenal atrophy. Abrupt withdrawal may therefore precipitate acute adrenal insufficiency (addisonian crisis). Patients who have been on prednisolone for longer than 3 weeks should have it withdrawn gradually.
* Glucocorticoids are normally secreted in increased amounts during physiological stress. As prolonged therapy with prednisolone leads to a diminished adrenocortical response, any significant injury (e.g. trauma, surgery) requires a temporary compensatory increase in the prednisolone dose.
* Prednisolone: increases gluconeogenesis; re-distributes fat to the face, neck and trunk, and causes protein breakdown in tissues such as skin, muscle and bone.

Related drugs
* Betamethasone, cortisone, dexamethasone, hydrocortisone, methylprednisolone, triamcinolone.

DIABETES AND ENDOCRINE SYSTEM

Management guidelines (pp. 125–127)
Diabetes mellitus
Complications of diabetes mellitus
Hyperthyroidism
Hypothyroidism

Drugs (pp. 128–136)
Carbimazole
Desmopressin
Gliptins
Glitazones
Glucagon-like peptide-1 (GLP-1) analogue
Insulin
Levothyroxine sodium
Metformin
Sulphonylureas

Management guidelines

DIABETES MELLITUS
- Regular exercise and education is important in both types of diabetes. Address other risk factors such as lipids, blood pressure control, smoking cessation and alcohol intake, if appropriate. Therapy should be tailored to the individual with regular multidisciplinary review.

Type 1 diabetes mellitus
- Insulin is always required (amount and type is tailored to the individual).
- Regular monitoring of blood glucose is required with appropriate adjustments in insulin dose.
- Patient compliance, education and self-management is essential to maintain optimal glucose levels and thus minimize the risk of long-term complications (i.e. retinopathy, peripheral neuropathy, nephropathy).

Type 2 diabetes mellitus
- Recommend diet therapy (reduce fat intake, increase intake of complex carbohydrates such as pasta and potatoes) and physical exercise.

The Hands–on Guide to Clinical Pharmacology, 3rd Edition. By S Chatu. Published 2010 by Blackwell Publishing Ltd.

- Oral hypoglycaemics are used when dietary measures have failed based on symptoms and HbA1c level.
- Sulphonylureas, metformin, acarbose and glitazones can be used alone or in combination.
- Metformin is the treatment of choice in patients not responding to diet (unless BMI <20 kg/m^2, in which case a sulphonylurea is the first choice).
- Newer agents called the gliptins (dipeptidyl peptidase 4 [DPP-4] inhibitors) and GLP-1 analogues can be added to metformin, sulphonylureas or glitazones to help achieve glycaemic control.
- Give insulin if HbA1c remains unacceptably high. Insulin can be added to oral hypoglycaemics or can substitute them.

COMPLICATIONS OF DIABETES MELLITUS
Hypoglycaemia
- In Type 1 diabetes this is usually due to a late meal, excessive exercise or inadequate carbohydrate intake; in type 2 diabetes hypoglycaemia is most commonly caused by inappropriate dosing of sulphonylurea drugs.
- If possible, give oral glucose in readily available form (e.g. dextrose tablets, sugary drink).
- If oral glucose not possible or no improvement after giving oral glucose, give glucagon 1 mg IM or IV but if still no response use 50–100 ml of 50% dextrose IV into large vein or use 10% dextrose but larger volumes required.
- Dextrose is irritant to veins. After giving IV dextrose, flush with 50 ml of normal saline.
- In malnourished individuals or in liver disease, giving glucagon is unlikely to correct hypoglycaemia because the liver is depleted of glycogen, which is converted to glucose.

Ketoacidosis
- Give IV fluids as usually severely dehydrated.
- Give insulin by IV infusion (sliding scale) until glucose levels are within normal range and arterial pH or venous bicarbonate has normalized.
- Monitor plasma potassium (administer potassium with IV fluids if in the normal range in order to prevent insulin-induced hypokalaemia).
- Insert nasogastric tube in comatose, vomiting and nauseated patients to prevent aspiration pneumonia.
- Give prophylactic heparin until patient is mobile (to prevent DVT).
- Change to subcutaneous insulin when the patient starts eating and has no ketones in urine.
- Investigate the cause of ketoacidosis; usually non-compliance with insulin, first presentation of type 1 diabetes or infection.

Hyperglycaemic hyperosmotic non-ketotic coma
- Usually presents in the elderly who have type 2 diabetes in the context of a MI, stroke or infection.
- Give IV fluids (use 0.45% saline if plasma Na$^+$ >150 mmol/L).
- Give treatment dose of heparin until patient is mobile (to prevent DVT).

- Give insulin as a sliding scale until glucose levels are within the normal range.
- Monitor plasma potassium (insulin causes hypokalaemia).
- Investigate the cause.

HYPERTHYROIDISM
- Control symptoms of hyperthyroidism with a beta blocker (e.g. propranolol) until euthyroid.
- Give an antithyroid agent: carbimazole or propylthiouracil.
- Oral radioactive iodine can be used as an alternative to antithyroid agents.
- Consider thyroidectomy in certain situations (e.g. cosmetic reasons, young women planning pregnancy).
- Patients often become hypothyroid after radioactive iodine or surgical treatment of hyperthyroidism. These patients then need to start thyroxine replacement therapy.
- *Thyrotoxic crisis*: give IV fluids, IV propranolol, IV hydrocortisone, oral carbimazole and then oral iodine; also supportive measures such as cooling with tepid sponging, paracetamol and treat any underlying infection.

HYPOTHYROIDISM
- Thyroxine replacement for life.
- Monitor thyroid function at regular intervals to ensure thyroid-stimulating hormone (TSH) is within the normal range.
- Can give IV liothyronine sodium for rapid response in myxoedema coma in conjunction with IV corticosteroids if pituitary hypothyroidism is suspected, e.g. no goitre, no history of radioiodine therapy and no thyroid surgery.

Drugs

CARBIMAZOLE

Class: Antithyroid drug

Indications
* Hyperthyroidism.

Mechanism of action
* Carbimazole decreases the production of thyroid hormones T3 (triiodothyronine) and T4 (thyroxine) in the thyroid gland.
* Carbimazole has several actions. The main action is blocking thyroid iodine trapping and inhibiting the enzyme thyroid peroxidase, which is necessary for thyroid hormone synthesis.
* Carbimazole also has a local immunosuppressive effect on the thyroid gland.

Adverse effects
* *Common*: GI disturbance, headache, rash, pruritus.
* *Rare*: bone marrow suppression (agranulocytosis, pancytopenia), jaundice, alopecia, arthralgia.

Contraindications
* None.
* Caution:
    * Breastfeeding.
    * Pregnancy (lowest dose possible should be used, as carbimazole in high dose crosses the placenta and can cause neonatal hypothyroidism or a goitre).
    * Hepatic impairment.

Interactions
* None.

Route of administration
* Oral.

Note
* Treatment of Graves' disease should continue for at least 1 year. Recurrence of hyperthyroidism occurs in more than half of the patients, but can be treated with another course of carbimazole.
* All patients must be advised to seek medical help if they develop features of bone marrow suppression (e.g. sore throat, mouth ulcers, bleeding). If a low neutrophil count is confirmed, treatment must be discontinued.
* Regular monitoring of thyroid function is essential. A TSH in the normal range reflects optimal dosing of carbimazole.
* Carbimazole can be replaced with propylthiouracil if adverse effects such as rash and itching cannot be tolerated.

Related drugs
* Propylthiouracil.

DESMOPRESSIN

Class: Synthetic antidiuretic hormone (ADH) analogue

Indications
- Treatment and diagnosis of pituitary diabetes insipidus.
- Primary nocturnal enuresis.
- To prevent bleeding in haemophilia and von Willebrand's disease.
- Postoperative polyuria/polydipsia, especially after neurosurgery.
- Post lumbar puncture headache.
- Test fibrinolytic response in Von Willebrand's disease.

Mechanism of action
- Desmopressin mimics the action of ADH.
- It selectively activates vasopressin$_2$ (V_2) receptors in renal tubular cells. This causes increased re-absorption of water and decreased excretion of sodium and water, thus controlling polyuria and polydipsia.
- In haemophilia and von Willebrand's disease, desmopressin increases the plasma concentration of factor VIII.

Adverse effects
- *Common*: dilutional hyponatraemia, fluid retention.
- *Rare*: hyponatraemic convulsions, abdominal pain, headache; epistaxis and nasal congestion with nasal spray.

Contraindications
- Psychogenic polydipsia.
- Polydipsia in alcohol dependence.
- Caution:
  - Renal impairment.
  - Heart failure.
  - Hypertension.

Interactions
- *Loperamide*: increased plasma concentration of oral desmopressin.
- *Indometacin*: potentiates the effects of desmopressin.

Route of administration
- Oral, intranasal, IM, IV, SC.

Note
- Desmopressin is used in the water deprivation test to differentiate between pituitary and nephrogenic diabetes insipidus.
- Doses of desmopressin should be adjusted to allow some diuresis in a 24-hour period. If dosing is excessive, there is a risk of hyponatraemia-induced convulsions.
- Vasopressin and terlipressin are used in the treatment of variceal bleeding (GI bleed) until definitive management is instigated. Desmopressin cannot be used since it has no vasoconstrictor effect.

Related drugs
- Terlipressin, vasopressin (ADH).

GLIPTINS

(Sitagliptin, vildagliptin)

Class: Gliptins (DPP-4 inhibitors)

Indications
* Type 2 diabetes in combination with other oral hypoglycaemics.

Mechanism of action
* Incretins are hormones produced by the gut, which increase in response to a meal. The main hormones, glucose-dependent insulinotropic polypeptide (GIP) and GLP-1, are involved in glucose regulation and stimulate insulin release from the pancreas. GLP-1 also inhibits glucagon release, thereby reducing liver glucose production. The enzyme DPP-4 breaks down incretins into inactive forms. Gliptins prevent hydrolysis of DPP-4, making it inactive and thereby enhancing levels of active incretin hormones.

Adverse effects
* *Common*: abdominal pain, nausea, vomiting – usually transient.
* *Rare*: peripheral oedema, nasopharyngitis, headache, dizziness, hypoglycaemia, (hepatitis – only with vildagliptin).

Contraindications
* Pregnancy.
* Breastfeeding.
* Ketoacidosis.

Interactions
* *Sulphonylureas*: concomitant use increases the risk of hypoglycaemia.

Route of administration
* Oral.

Note
* Gliptins are weight neutral.
* Increased risk of hypoglycaemia with sulphonylureas, hence lower doses of sulphonylureas should be considered.
* Gliptins can cause significant reductions in the HbA1c level.

GLITAZONES

(Rosiglitazone, pioglitazone)

Class: Thiazolidinediones

Indications
* Type 2 diabetes (monotherapy or in combination with other oral hypoglycaemics).

Mechanism of action
* These drugs act on peroxisome proliferator-activated receptor gamma (PPAR gamma) receptors in skeletal muscle, adipose tissue and the liver increasing insulin sensitivity and thereby reducing plasma glucose.

Adverse effects
* *Common*: weight gain, fluid retention.
* *Rare*: hepatitis, osteoporosis.

Contraindications
* Established cardiovascular disease or PVD (only rosiglitazone is contraindicated).
* Heart failure.
* Pregnancy and breastfeeding.
* Hepatic impairment.

Interactions
* None.

Route of administration
* Oral.

Note
* Rosiglitazone has limited use as it is contraindicated in cardiovascular disease, which is a common problem in type 2 diabetes.
* The beneficial effects of glitazones can take up to 6–8 weeks to establish.

GLUCAGON-LIKE PEPTIDE 1 (GLP-1) ANALOGUE

(Exenatide, liraglutide)

Class: Incretin hormone analogue

Indications
* Type 2 diabetes in combination with other oral hypoglycaemics.

Mechanism of action
* The incretin effect is diminished in type 2 diabetes. There is a deficiency of GLP-1 and resistance to GIP. Replacing the incretin hormone GLP-1, which is not inactivated by DPP-4, results in:
  * Insulin secretion from the pancreas.
  * Inhibition of glucagon release from the pancreas.
  * Delays gastric emptying thereby reducing glucose absorption into the circulation and causes early satiety.

Adverse effects
* *Common*: nausea, satiety.
* *Rare*: pancreatitis, nasopharyngitis, headache, dizziness, hyperhidrosis.

Contraindications
* Ketoacidosis.
* Pregnancy.
* Breastfeeding.

Interactions
* None.

Route of administration
* SC.

Note
* Exenatide causes a beneficial reduction in blood pressure.
* Antibodies can develop to exenatide, but the clinical relevance of this is uncertain.
* Usually sulphonylureas are stopped or the dose reduced due to increased risk of hypoglycaemia with GLP-1 analogues.
* GLP-1 analogues have been shown to cause significant weight reduction in patients with type 2 diabetes.
* GLP-1 analogues can be used in combination with insulin to help reduce weight and thus insulin requirements.

INSULIN

Class: Peptide hormone

Indications

- Diabetes mellitus types 1 and 2.
- Ketoacidosis.
- Hyperglycaemic hyperosmotic non-ketotic coma.
- Emergency treatment of hyperkalaemia (IV glucose must be co-administered).

Mechanism of action

- Insulin lowers plasma glucose concentration by:
  1. Stimulating glucose transport into fat and muscle cells.
  2. Stimulating the liver to store glucose in the form of glycogen.
  3. Inhibiting gluconeogenesis, lipolysis and protein breakdown.

Adverse effects

- *Common*: hypoglycaemia, weight gain.
- *Rare*: fat hypertrophy or atrophy at the injection site (sites should be rotated), rash, pruritus.

Contraindications

- Hypoglycaemia.

Interactions

- *Alcohol*: this enhances the hypoglycaemic effect.
- *Beta blockers*: these mask the warning signs of hypoglycaemia; they also enhance the hypoglycaemic effect.

Route of administration

- SC (deliver via pen injector devices, syringe and needle, or as continuous infusion), IM, IV.

Note

- There are five different types of insulin preparations:
  - Quick-acting insulin analogues (insulin lispro, insulin aspart) – immediate onset, duration of action 4–6 hours.
  - Short-acting insulin (soluble insulin) – onset 30 minutes, duration of action up to 8 hours.
  - Intermediate-acting insulin (isophane insulin) – duration of action 14–22 hours.
  - Long-acting insulin (e.g. crystalline insulin zinc suspension) – duration of action 36 hours; and long-acting insulin analogue (glargine) – duration of action 24 hours.
  - Mixed (short-acting with intermediate-acting insulin or analogues).
- Stress, infection, trauma, pregnancy and puberty can increase insulin requirements.
- Insulin promotes the influx of potassium, as well as glucose, into cells. As a consequence, the plasma potassium concentration can drop to dangerously low levels, particularly during insulin treatment of ketoacidosis. In this situation IV potassium must be given.
- Different regimes are adapted to the individual. Common regimes are a dose of short-acting insulin 15–30 minutes prior to meals and intermediate-acting insulin at bedtime; or a mixed preparation twice daily (intermediate with short-acting).

LEVOTHYROXINE SODIUM

Class: Thyroid hormone

Indications
- Hypothyroidism.

Mechanism of action
- Levothyroxine sodium replaces and mimics endogenous thyroxine. Thyroxine is required to regulate many of the body's metabolic functions.

Adverse effects
- *Rare*: cardiac dysrhythmias, tachycardia, angina pain, restlessness, sweating, weight loss (all with excessive doses).

Contraindications
- Thyrotoxicosis.

Interactions
- *Antiepileptics (carbamazepine, phenytoin)*: increase the metabolism of levothyroxine.
- *Rifampicin*: increases the metabolism of levothyroxine.
- *Warfarin*: levothyroxine increases the effect of warfarin.

Route of administration
- Oral.

Note
- Plasma TSH levels should be monitored to assess treatment. TSH levels may take up to 10 weeks to return to normal after optimum thyroxine levels are achieved.
- Levothyroxine should be introduced gradually in patients with IHD, as it can cause excessive cardiac stimulation (consider a pretherapy ECG).
- In patients with diabetes requiring thyroxine, the dose of insulin or oral hypoglycaemics may have to be increased.

Related drugs
- Liothyronine sodium (faster acting than levothyroxine sodium).

METFORMIN

Class: Biguanide

Indications
* Type 2 diabetes mellitus.

Mechanism of action
* Metformin requires the presence of insulin as it is principally an insulin-sensitizing agent. It does not influence insulin release.
* Metformin increases peripheral glucose utilization and decreases gluconeogenesis, possibly through its action on membrane phospholipids.
* It also inhibits glucose absorption from the intestinal lumen.
* Metformin has non-glycaemic benefits that reduce mortality in type 2 diabetes.

Adverse effects
* *Common*: anorexia, nausea, vomiting, abdominal pain, diarrhoea.
* *Rare*: lactic acidosis (especially in renal impairment), reduced vitamin B_{12} absorption, metallic taste, hepatitis.

Contraindications
* Pregnancy.
* Breastfeeding.
* *Note*: metformin is also contraindicated in the following conditions, since they predispose to lactic acidosis:
  * Conditions that may cause tissue hypoxia (e.g. respiratory failure, sepsis, severe heart failure).
  * Hepatic or renal impairment (if creatinine 150 umol/l or more).
  * Severe dehydration.

Interactions
* *Alcohol*: excessive alcohol intake with metformin can predispose to lactic acidosis.

Route of administration
* Oral.

Note
* Metformin does not cause hypoglycaemia, unlike sulphonylureas.
* It is used in type 2 diabetes mellitus patients, alone or in combination with other oral hypoglycaemics and/or insulin.
* Metformin reduces appetite, thus encouraging weight loss. It is therefore the treatment of choice in obese diabetics.
* Metformin should be stopped prior to receiving iodine-containing X-ray contrast, in order to prevent renal impairment. It should also be stopped prior to general anaesthesia as there is a risk of lactic acidosis. It can be restarted after the procedure if renal function is normal.

SULPHONYLUREAS

(Gliclazide, glibenclamide, glimepiride, glipizide, tolbutamide)

Class: Sulphonylurea

Indications
* Type 2 diabetes mellitus.

Mechanism of action
* These drugs stimulate insulin secretion by binding to sulphonylurea receptors and blocking ATP-dependent potassium channels in pancreatic beta cells. This causes depolarization and insulin release.
* They also inhibit gluconeogenesis.

Adverse effects
* *Common*: hypoglycaemia, weight gain.
* *Rare*: GI disturbance, bone marrow suppression, rash, hepatitis.

Contraindications
* Acute porphyria.
* Ketoacidosis.
* Pregnancy.
* Breastfeeding.
* Caution:
  * The elderly and patients with hepatic or renal impairment are very susceptible to hypoglycaemia.

Interactions
* *Corticosteroids*: antagonize the hypoglycaemic effect of gliclazide.
* *Loop diuretics, thiazides*: antagonize the hypoglycaemic effect.

Route of administration
* Oral.

Note
* The types of sulphonylureas differ in terms of duration of action.
* Sulphonylureas are often combined with metformin in those who cannot achieve adequate glycaemic control. They can also be combined with acarbose, gliptins, glitazones, and GLP-1 analogues.
* As sulphonylureas do not provide adequate glycaemic control during surgery, pregnancy and illness (e.g. infection, MI, trauma), they are usually temporarily substituted with insulin for these events.

DERMATOLOGY

Management guidelines (pp. 137–138)
Acne
Atopic eczema
Psoriasis
Rosacea

Drugs (pp. 139–142)
Calcitriol
Chlorpheniramine
Dithranol
Isotretinoin

Management guidelines

ACNE
- Aim of treatment is to remove the blockage of pilar drainage (comedones) and to treat the infection.
- Consider psychological impact on the patient.
- Ensure good skin hygiene before initiating treatment.
  - Mild acne:
    - Topical antibiotics – erythromycin, clindamycin.
    - Benzoyl peroxide gel.
    - Topical isotretinoin (used in comedonal and papulopustular acne).
    - Note: combinations of the above are most effective.
  - Moderate acne:
    - As for mild acne plus oral antibiotics (minocycline), or in females oral oestrogen with cyproterone acetate (antiandrogen).
  - Severe acne:
    - Oral isotretinoin if the above fails.

ATOPIC ECZEMA
- Identify and remove any causative agents (e.g. bleaches, soaps, detergents).
- Topical and systemic agents can be used in various combinations and should be tailored to the individual:
  - *Topical treatment* (for mild to moderate eczema):
    - Unscented emollients – used on skin and supplemented with bath or shower emollients (soap substitutes).

The Hands–on Guide to Clinical Pharmacology, 3rd Edition. By S Chatu.
Published 2010 by Blackwell Publishing Ltd.

- Bandages containing ichthammol and zinc are sometimes used over topical corticosteroids or emollients for treatment of eczema involving the limbs.
- Corticosteroids are often used; potency of the preparation depends on the site and severity of the condition.
- Antibiotics for superimposed infections.
- *Note*: Topical tacrolimus or pimecrolimus can be used if resistant to or unable to tolerate topical steroids.
- *Systemic treatment* (for moderate to severe eczema): as above plus any of the following:
  - Antihistamines to reduce itching (e.g. chlorpheniramine).
  - Ultraviolet B (UVB) phototherapy.
  - Psoralen with ultraviolet A (PUVA) radiation.
  - Corticosteroids (only used temporarily in severe intractable eczema).
  - Consider immunosuppressants (ciclosporin or azathioprine) if other treatment options fail.
  - Antibiotics for superimposed infections.

PSORIASIS

- Topical and systemic agents can be used in various combinations and should be tailored to the individual:
  - *Topical treatment* (for mild to moderate psoriasis):
    - Emollients.
    - Calcitriol or calcipotriol ointment.
    - Corticosteroid.
    - Coal tar.
    - Dithranol cream.
    - Tazarotene (a retinoid).
  - *Systemic treatment* (for moderate to severe psoriasis):
    - PUVA radiation.
    - UVB phototherapy.
    - Retinoid (e.g. acitretin).
    - Methotrexate.
    - Ciclosporin.
    - Biological therapies, e.g. adalimumab, etanercept, infliximab.

ROSACEA

- Avoid precipitants (e.g. hot drinks, alcohol, spicy foods).
- Treatment may be:
  - *Topical* – metronidazole, or sodium sulfacetamide with 5% sulphur.
  - *Systemic* – tetracycline or minocycline, or isotretinoin if antibiotics fail.
- Facial flushing can be treated with:
  - Propranolol or clonidine.
  - Cosmetic camouflage.
  - Laser treatment.
- Surgery may be required for complications such as rhinophyma.

Drugs

CALCITRIOL

Class: Vitamin D analogue

Indications
* Psoriasis (topical use only).
* Hypocalcaemia (e.g. in chronic renal failure, hypoparathyroidism, malabsorption).
* Postmenopausal osteoporosis.

Mechanism of action
* Calcitriol is 1,25-dihydroxycholecalciferol, a synthetic hydroxylated form of vitamin D.
* In psoriasis, calcitriol acts by inhibiting fibroblast, lymphocyte and keratinocyte proliferation.
* In hypocalcaemia, calcitriol raises serum calcium by:
   1. Stimulating absorption of calcium in the GI tract.
   2. Increasing calcium re-absorption in the kidneys, thereby reducing its excretion.
   3. Stimulating calcium release from bones.

Adverse effects
* *Common*: skin irritation and itching with topical use; nausea, vomiting, polyuria, diarrhoea, vertigo and weakness with systemic overdose.

Contraindications
* Hypercalcaemia.
* Calcifications secondary to metastases.

Interactions
* *Thiazide diuretics*: concomitant use increases the risk of hypercalcaemia.

Route of administration
* Oral, IV, topical.

Note
* Topical calcitriol should be avoided in children and on the face, owing to irritant effects on the skin.
* Unlike dithranol or tar preparations for psoriasis, topical calcitriol does not smell or stain. It also does not involve the risk of skin atrophy that is associated with topical steroids.
* A total of 90% of the body's vitamin D comes from sunlight exposure, the remaining 10% is dietary (cod liver oil, fatty fish, fortified milk and cereals).
* People not exposed to sunlight are prone to vitamin D deficiency (e.g. housebound elderly).

Related drugs
* Systemic formulations: alfacalcidol (1 alpha-cholecalciferol), cholecalciferol (vitamin D_3), dihydrotachysterol, ergocalciferol (vitamin D_2).
* Topical formulations: calcipotriol, tacalcitol.

CHLORPHENIRAMINE

Class: Histamine$_1$ (H$_1$)-receptor antagonist

Indications
- Allergic reactions (e.g. urticaria, hay fever).
- Anaphylaxis.

Mechanism of action
- Chlorpheniramine blocks the action of histamine which is released from mast cells and basophils in response to an allergic reaction, by binding to H$_1$ receptors, in blood vessels, respiratory tract and the GI tract. This inhibitory action alleviates symptoms of allergy such as sneezing, itching, swelling and watery eyes.

Adverse effects
- *Common*: antimuscarinic effects (e.g. blurred vision, urinary retention, dry mouth), dizziness, nausea, drowsiness.
- *Rare*: palpitations, hepatic dysfunction, tachycardia, paradoxical CNS stimulation.

Contraindications
- None.
- Caution:
  - BPH.
  - Glaucoma.
  - Urinary retention.
  - Hepatic impairment.

Interactions
- *TCAs*: muscarinic and sedative effects are enhanced.
- *Alcohol*: sedative effects are enhanced.

Route of administration
- Oral, IM, SC, IV.

Note
- Chlorpheniramine is less sedating than other 'older' antihistamines in its group.
- Newer antihistamines are non-sedating (see below).
- Patients should be warned about the possible sedating effects. This is particularly important if driving is involved.
- Drowsiness tends to improve after a few days' use of chlorpheniramine.

Related drugs
- Other sedating antihistamines: brompheniramine, clemastine, cyproheptadine, diphenhydramine, doxylamine, hydroxyzine, promethazine, trimeprazine.
- Non-sedating antihistamines: cetirizine, desloratadine, fexofenadine, levocetirizine, loratadine, mizolastine, terfenadine.

DITHRANOL

Class: Anthraquinone derivative

Indications
* Chronic psoriasis.

Mechanism of action
* Dithranol is 1,8,9-trihydroxyanthranol, also known as anthralin.
* Dithranol decreases mitotic activity and DNA synthesis in the hyperplastic epidermal layer of the skin. This results in normalization of epidermal cell proliferation and keratinization. The end result is inhibition of skin cell growth that occurs in psoriasis.

Adverse effects
* *Common*: irritation of unaffected skin, staining of skin, hair, nails or clothes/bed sheets.
* *Rare*: rash.

Contraindications
* Acute psoriasis.
* Pustular psoriasis.

Interactions
* None known.

Route of administration
* Topical.

Note
* Dithranol should be stopped temporarily in acute flare-ups of psoriasis.
* It should not be used on the face, genitalia or flexures (too irritant).
* To reduce staining, the patient should wear gloves when applying dithranol. When applied at bedtime, old pyjamas should be worn and old bed sheets used.
* Skin irritation caused by accidentally applying dithranol to non-affected skin around a psoriasis plaque can be relieved by applying zinc oxide.
* Treatment with dithranol is usually under the supervision of a dermatologist.

ISOTRETINOIN

Class: Retinoid

Indications
- Acne (especially severe acne and acne not responding to systemic antibiotics).

Mechanism of action
- Exact mechanism is not fully understood.
- It inhibits sebaceous gland function and thereby reduces sebum production.
- Isotretinoin also reduces production of keratin in the outer layer of the skin.
- In addition, isotretinoin has some anti-inflammatory properties.

Adverse effects
- *Common*: dry mucous membranes and skin, photosensitivity, alopecia.
- *Rare*: hypertriglyceridaemia, visual disturbances, benign intracranial hypertension, hepatitis, mood changes, hearing impairment, blood disorders.

Contraindications
- Pregnancy.
- Breastfeeding.
- Renal impairment.
- Hepatic impairment.
- Hypertriglyceridaemia.
- Hypervitaminosis A.

Interactions
- *Vitamin A*: concomitant use may lead to hypervitaminosis A (stomatitis, dry nose, epistaxis, pruritus).
- *Tetracyclines* (*doxycycline, minocycline, tetracycline*): concomitant use may predispose to benign intracranial hypertension.

Route of administration
- Oral, topical

Note
- Isotretinoin should only be prescribed by specialists.
- Regular monitoring of lipids and liver function is essential.
- Retinoids can cause dryness of mucous membranes leading to intolerance of contact lenses.
- Isotretinoin is teratogenic. Women must be advised to avoid pregnancy while taking isotretinoin, and contraception must be used 1 month before, during and after treatment.

Related drugs
- Acitretin, tretinoin.

PAIN MANAGEMENT

Management guidelines

GENERAL PRINCIPLES OF PAIN CONTROL WITH ANALGESICS

Analgesics are usually divided into two main groups:
* Primary (non-specific) analgesics, which can be subdivided into:
    * Simple analgesics: *paracetamol, NSAIDs*.
    * Opioid analgesics:
        ◦ *Weak opioids*: codeine phosphate, tramadol, dihydrocodeine, co-dydramol, co-codamol.
        ◦ *Strong opioids*: morphine, diamorphine, pethidine, fentanyl, buprenorphine, methadone.
* Secondary (specific) analgesics:
    * These medications provide analgesia by removing the cause of pain (e.g. GTN spray in angina, omeprazole in gastric ulcer).

Analgesic ladder
* If there is no treatable cause of pain, use the analgesic ladder for symptomatic pain relief.
* Start at the appropriate step with regular review:
    * Step 1: paracetamol +/- NSAID.

The Hands–on Guide to Clinical Pharmacology, 3rd Edition. By S Chatu.
Published 2010 by Blackwell Publishing Ltd.

- Step 2: weak opioid (e.g. codeine phosphate, tramadol) + paracetamol +/- NSAID.
- Step 3: strong opioid (e.g. morphine, fentanyl) + paracetamol +/- NSAID.
- Inadequate analgesia requires a move to the next step, rather than to another drug of similar efficacy after maximum dose and an adequate time period has been allowed for the medication to be effective.
- Adjuvant medication should be prescribed at any stage; antidotes for common side-effects, e.g. antiemetics for nausea, laxatives for constipation, PPIs with NSAIDs if history of peptic ulcer. Amitriptyline for neuropathic pain and bisphosphonates for bone pain from metastatic malignancy.

ALTERNATIVE METHODS OF PAIN CONTROL
- Psychological care (e.g. explanation of pain, re-assurance).
- Hot or cold applications (e.g. hot water bottle, ice pack).
- Immobilization with collars, splints, corsets, etc.
- Acupuncture.
- Transcutaneous electrical nerve stimulation (TENS).
- Nerve block using local anaesthetic.

BONE PAIN
- Treat any underlying cause; a common cause is metastatic malignancy.
- Follow analgesic ladder, but NSAIDs are particularly effective.
- Radiotherapy is effective in metastatic bone pain.
- Calcitonin, bisphosphonates or opioids may also be used.
- Surgery to stabilize weakened or fractured bone with rods, plates or screws.

MUSCLE SPASM PAIN
- Treat any underlying cause.
- *Smooth muscle spasm*:
  - Typically experienced in renal colic or intestinal colic e.g. irritable bowel syndrome.
  - Give hyoscine butylbromide, a smooth muscle relaxant.
  - Stronger analgesia (e.g. opioids) may be required.
- *Skeletal muscle spasm*:
  - May be experienced in multiple sclerosis, spinal cord injury or other trauma.
  - The following agents may be used:
    ○ Baclofen, a skeletal muscle relaxant that acts centrally and on the spinal cord.
    ○ Diazepam, which acts on GABA receptors in the CNS.
    ○ Dantrolene, which acts peripherally on skeletal muscle.
  - *Note*: Above medications should not be used for muscular spasm caused by minor injuries.
  - *Nocturnal leg cramps*:
    ○ Quinine can be used long term. It reduces the frequency of cramps by roughly 25%.
    ○ Effect may not be apparent for up to 4 weeks.

◦ Treatment should be interrupted every 3 months to assess the need for continuing therapy.

NEUROPATHIC PAIN

* Common causes are diabetic neuropathy, post stroke, spinal cord injury.
* Treat initially with antidepressant (amitriptyline) or anticonvulsant (carbamazepine).
* If these are ineffective or inappropriate, consider gabapentin, pregabalin, local lidocaine gel.
* Opioids are only partially effective in neuropathic pain. Consider these when other treatment options have failed.
* TENS and acupuncture may be effective in some patients.
* Surgery may be an option in some cases.
* If refractory to above, refer for specialist advice for consideration of second-line anticonvulsants (sodium valproate, lamotrigine), SSRIs, ketamine, topical capsaicin, opioids, neuromodulation with pulsed radiofrequency to damage nerves and steroid injection into the nerves.

Drug types

NON-STEROIDAL ANTI-INFLAMMATORY DRUGS (NSAIDS)
Types of NSAIDs
1. Salicylic acids: aspirin.
2. Propionic acids: ibuprofen, naproxen.
3. Acetic acids: indometacin.
4. Fenamates: mefenamic acid.
5. Pyrazolones: phenylbutazone.
6. Phenylacetic acids: diclofenac.
7. Oxicams: meloxicam, piroxicam, tenoxicam.
8. COX-2 inhibitors: celecoxib, etodolac, etoricoxib.

Indications
- Inflammatory diseases (e.g. rheumatoid arthritis).
- Pain (especially musculoskeletal pain).
- Perioperative analgesia (alongside opioids and local anaesthetics – concept known as 'balanced analgesia').

Mechanism of action
- NSAIDs act through reversible inhibition of enzymes COX-1 and COX-2, which results in decreased conversion of arachidonic acid to prostaglandins, which have pathological (pro- inflammatory) and physiological functions.
- Aspirin differs in the fact that it irreversibly inhibits COX-1 and COX-2. It also has an antiplatelet effect.
- COX-2 inhibitors specifically target COX-2.
- The desired pharmacological effects of NSAIDs are thought to be due to the inhibition of COX-2, which is inducible in inflammatory conditions and leads to the production of inflammatory cytokines.

Adverse effects
- These are mainly related to the inhibition of COX-1 (expressed in most tissues and maintains physiological processes) and include:
  - GI disturbances (peptic ulcer, gastritis).
  - Bleeding (with aspirin).
  - Bronchoconstriction.
  - Renal impairment.

OPIOID ANALGESICS
Indications
- Pain is the main indication (morphine or diamorphine are most commonly used in severe pain).
- Other uses:
  - Acute pulmonary oedema secondary to heart failure (morphine or diamorphine).

- Diarrhoea (codeine).
- Cough (codeine or dihydrocodeine).
- Methadone is used to prevent withdrawal symptoms in opioid abusers.

Mechanism of action
- Opioid analgesics mimic endogenous opioids by acting on mu, delta and kappa opioid receptors in the spinal cord and in areas of the brainstem that are rich in naturally occurring opioids:
    - Full agonists: codeine, dextropropoxyphene, diamorphine, dihydrocodeine, fentanyl, morphine, pethidine.
    - Partial agonists: buprenorphine, pentazocine, tramadol.

Adverse effects
- Respiratory depression (with high doses).
- Constipation.
- Nausea and vomiting.
- Hypotension, rash, itching (due to histamine release).
- Dependence and tolerance (dependence very rarely occurs when used correctly for pain).

Opioid antagonists
- These are used to reverse severe or unwanted opioid effects, which usually occur after overdose:
    - Naloxone (rapidly acting).
    - Naltrexone (longer duration of action).

Note
- Codeine is commonly used as a weaker alternative to morphine.
- Opioid antagonists or abrupt withdrawal of an opioid can precipitate a withdrawal syndrome. This typically becomes evident after about 12 hours. It can include symptoms such as yawning, sweating and rhinorrhoea, followed by irritability, insomnia, tremor and gooseflesh ('cold turkey' effect). Symptoms reach a peak 2–3 days after withdrawal and recede after about 1 week. Diarrhoea, vomiting and abdominal cramps may also occur.

Drugs

CO-CODAMOL, CO-DYDRAMOL

Class: Compound analgesics

Indications
*   Moderate pain.

Mechanism of action
*   The paracetamol component inhibits production of chemical mediators that cause pain (see Paracetamol).
*   The codeine and dihydrocodeine components act by binding to opioid receptors in the CNS to decrease pain (see Morphine).

Adverse effects
*   *Common*: nausea, vomiting, constipation, drowsiness.
*   *Rare*: rash, euphoria.

Contraindications
*   None.
*   Caution:
    *   Chronic respiratory disease.
    *   Elderly.

Interactions
*   See Morphine, Paracetamol (pp. 149 and 151).

Route of administration
*   Oral.

Note
*   Overdose can be hazardous with combination products as the opioid component may cause respiratory depression and the paracetamol may lead to liver damage.
*   Co-codamol is available in different strengths, i.e. the dose of codeine varies.
*   There are combined products available combining aspirin with paracetamol.

MORPHINE

Class: Opioid analgesic

Indications
- Severe pain (e.g. MI, perioperative analgesia, pain in terminal illness).
- Acute pulmonary oedema secondary to heart failure.
- Intractable cough in terminal care.

Mechanism of action
- Morphine mimics endogenous opioids by acting on mu, delta and kappa opioid receptors in the spinal cord and in areas of the brainstem that are rich in naturally occurring opioids.
- Opioids have an analgesic, anxiolytic and euphoric effect.
- In pulmonary oedema, morphine reduces preload by dilating large veins and in conjunction with its anxiolytic effect improves breathlessness.

Adverse effects
- *Common*: nausea, vomiting, drowsiness, constipation; respiratory depression and hypotension with larger doses.
- *Rare*: hallucinations, difficulty with micturition, dry mouth, urticaria, biliary spasm, mood changes.

Contraindications
- Acute respiratory depression.
- Raised intracranial pressure (morphine may interfere with neurological assessment).
- Head injury (morphine may interfere with neurological assessment).
- Phaeochromocytoma.
- Acute alcohol intoxication.
- Paralytic ileus.

Interactions
- *Alcohol*: enhances the sedative and hypotensive effects of morphine.
- *Hypnotics*: enhance the sedative and hypotensive effects of morphine.

Route of administration
- IM, IV, oral, rectal, SC.

Note
- The effects of morphine can be reversed with naloxone, a rapidly acting opioid antagonist.
- Tolerance to morphine begins to emerge after about 2 weeks of continuous administration. Subsequently, the dose should be increased.
- Abrupt withdrawal of morphine results in a withdrawal syndrome (e.g. myalgia, sweating, yawning).
- Pethidine and alfentanil are used for pain relief during endoscopic procedures owing to their short duration of action.

Related drugs
- Buprenorphine, codeine, dihydrocodeine, diamorphine, alfentanil, fentanyl, methadone, oxycodone, pethidine, remifentanil, tramadol.

NON-STEROIDAL ANTI-INFLAMMATORY DRUGS (NSAIDs)

Ibuprofen, diclofenac, indometacin, naproxen

Class: NSAID

Indications
- Mild to moderate pain, especially associated with inflammation, e.g. musculoskeletal and postoperative pain.

Mechanism of action
- NSAIDs are potent inhibitors of the enzymes COX-1 and COX-2. This leads to inhibition of prostaglandin synthesis and hence to:
  - A decrease in vascular permeability and vasodilatation (anti-inflammatory effect).
  - A decrease in sensitization of pain afferents (analgesic effect).
  - A decrease in the effect of prostaglandins on the hypothalamus (antipyretic effect).

Adverse effects
- *Common*: nausea, diarrhoea, epigastric discomfort, peptic ulcers, gastritis.
- *Rare*: bronchospasm, renal failure, fluid retention, gluteal abscess (when diclofenac injected IM).

Contraindications
- Active peptic ulceration.
- Severe cardiac failure.
- Pregnancy and breastfeeding.
- Caution:
  - Renal, hepatic and cardiac impairment.
  - Asthma.
  - Coagulation defects.

Interactions
- *Corticosteroids*: increased risk of peptic ulceration when NSAIDs are given with corticosteroids.

Route of administration
- IM, IV, oral, rectal, topical.

Note
- Clinically NSAIDs are used in postoperative pain, acute gout, other musculoskeletal pain and ureteric colic.
- NSAIDs do not cause respiratory depression, dependence or impaired GI motility.
- IM or rectal diclofenac has a comparable effect to pethidine in the management of ureteric colic.
- Diclofenac topical gel is effective in the treatment of actinic keratosis. In this instance it should be continued for 2–3 months.
- NSAIDs can cause exacerbation of asthma and inflammatory bowel disease in some patients.
- Those at risk of peptic ulcers or with a history should receive either a COX-2 inhibitor or a NSAID with gastroprotective treatment e.g. omeprazole.

PARACETAMOL

Class: Non-opioid analgesic and antipyretic

Indications
*   Mild to moderate pain.
*   Pyrexia.

Mechanism of action
*   Paracetamol is a weak inhibitor of both COX-1 and COX-2, which are responsible for the production of prostaglandins and thromboxane.
*   Paracetamol may also act through selective inhibition of COX-3, a more recently discovered enzyme found in the brain and spinal cord.
*   It is believed that these actions and other possible unknown mechanisms result in its analgesic and antipyretic effect.

Adverse effects
*   *Rare*: rash leucopenia, thrombocytopenia.

Contraindications
*   None.
*   Caution:
    *   Hepatic impairment.
    *   Renal impairment.
    *   Chronic alcohol abuse.

Interactions
*   No serious interactions.

Route of administration
*   Oral, rectal, IV.

Note
*   Paracetamol has similar analgesic efficacy to aspirin. As paracetamol does not cause gastric irritation it is preferred to aspirin for pain relief, especially in the elderly.
*   Paracetamol is commonly used in children, as it is not associated with Reye's syndrome (unlike aspirin).
*   Paracetamol is effective in musculoskeletal pain. Opioids are preferred in visceral pain.
*   Toxic metabolites of paracetamol are generated more rapidly when administered with drugs that induce hepatic enzymes (e.g. rifampicin) leading to possible liver damage at therapeutic doses.
*   *N*-acetylcysteine is an effective antidote in paracetamol overdose (see p. 220).

PETHIDINE

Class: Opioid analgesic

Indications
* Moderate to severe pain (e.g. perioperatively, labour). Pain relief during medical procedures e.g. colonoscopy

Mechanism of action
* Pethidine acts by stimulating mu, delta and kappa opioid receptors in the spinal cord and in areas of the brainstem that are rich in naturally occurring opioids.
* It creates a sense of euphoria, which contributes to the analgesic effect by reducing anxiety and stress.

Adverse effects
* *Common*: nausea, vomiting, constipation, drowsiness, dizziness, confusion.
* *Rare*: shortness of breath, convulsions in overdose.

Contraindications
* Severe renal impairment.
* Respiratory failure.
* Alcoholism.
* Concomitant use of MAOIs.

Interactions
* *Cimetidine*: this inhibits metabolism of pethidine and thus increases its plasma concentration.
* *MAOIs*: concomitant use with pethidine can cause CNS excitation or CNS depression.

Route of administration
* Oral, IM, IV, SC.

Note
* Owing to its lipid solubility, pethidine has a rapid onset of action. It is a less potent analgesic than morphine.
* Pethidine can be used in labour, as adverse effects on the baby are less pronounced than with other opioids (due to its short half-life of 2–4 hours), and also because it does not inhibit uterine contractions. However, pethidine may cause respiratory depression in the neonate if given to the labouring mother.
* Larger doses of pethidine are required if given orally due to extensive first-pass metabolism.
* Unlike morphine, pethidine does not cause pupillary constriction in overdose. Naloxone is an effective antidote in pethidine overdose.
* Pethidine is less constipating than morphine.
* Norpethidine, a metabolite of pethidine, may accumulate and cause convulsions by stimulating the CNS. This is more likely in renal impairment.

Related drugs
* Diamorphine, fentanyl, methadone, morphine.

INFECTION

The Hands–on Guide to Clinical Pharmacology, 3rd Edition. By S Chatu.
Published 2010 by Blackwell Publishing Ltd.

Tetracycline, trimethoprim
Vancomycin
Zidovudine

Management guidelines

CLOSTRIDIUM DIFFICILE INFECTION

* Treat with oral metronidazole for 10 days and stop all other antibiotics if possible.
* If symptoms are not improving or worsening, start oral vancomycin (sometimes high doses required or a pulsed regime).
* Give IV metronidazole if oral treatment inappropriate (or give oral medication via nasogastric tube).
* In those not responding to conventional treatment, consider oral rifampicin, IV immunoglobulin or teicoplanin.

CONJUNCTIVITIS (INFECTIVE)

* Usually caused by *Staphylococcus aureus, Streptococcus pneumoniae, Haemophilus influenzae* or adenoviruses.
* Most cases are self-resolving. If treatment is desired, give chloramphenicol eye drops or ointment (this covers all the aforementioned pathogens except adenovirus, for which there is no treatment available). Remember to treat both eyes (cross-infection is common).
* In allergic conjunctivitis, give sodium cromoglycate or antihistamine eye drops.

HUMAN IMMUNODEFICIENCY VIRUS (HIV) AND OPPORTUNISTIC INFECTIONS

* There is no cure for HIV, but the aim of treatment is to reduce viral load and thereby increase the CD4 cell count (T_4 'helper' cells).
* Treatment for HIV must be under specialist supervision or undertaken by a doctor with experience in the field.
* Apart from antiretroviral therapy, the patient may also be on treatment for opportunistic infections such as cytomegalovirus (CMV) retinitis or *Pneumocystis jiroveci* (*P. carinii*) pneumonia.
* Three categories of antiretroviral agents used in HIV are available:

    1. *Nucleoside analogue reverse transcriptase inhibitors* (NRTIs): abacavir, didanosine, emtricitabine, lamivudine, stavudine, tenofovir, zidovudine.

    2. *Non-nucleoside reverse transcriptase inhibitors* (non-NRTIs): efavirenz, nevirapine.

    3. *Protease inhibitors*: amprenavir, indinavir, lopinavir, nelfinavir, ritonavir, saquinavir.

* Treatment is usually two NRTIs with a protease inhibitor, or two NRTIs with a non-NRTI. However, these regimes are subject to frequent updates and changes.
* Other drugs used in resistant cases are *enfuvirtide* (fusion inhibitor), *maraviroc* (used in those with CCR5-tropic HIV) and *raltegravir* (inhibitor of HIV integrase).

Common opportunistic infections
- *Pneumocystis jiroveci* (*P. carinii*) pneumonia:
  - Co-trimoxazole given orally or IV, depending on the severity of infection is used first-line.
  - Atovaquone, combination of clindamycin + primaquine, or pentamidine are considered if co-trimoxazole is intolerable or contra-indicated.
  - Adjuvant corticosteroids should be started in conjunction with above therapy, or within 72 hours if there is associated hypoxia, in order to reduce risk of respiratory failure.
- Cerebral toxoplasmosis:
  - Pyrimethamine and sulfadiazine in combination.
- Cryptococcal meningitis:
  - Amphotericin B + flucytosine usually for 2 weeks.
- CMV retinitis:
  - Ganciclovir, cidofovir or foscarnet used IV; alternatively use oral valganciclovir.

INFECTIVE ENDOCARDITIS
- Detailed guidelines exist and consultation with a cardiologist or microbiologist is recommended.

Prophylaxis
- Prophylaxis is no longer necessary in patients with cardiac abnormalities (e.g. congenital defects, valvular heart disease, artificial heart valves) and other high-risk groups (e.g. previous infective endocarditis) undergoing dental, surgical or other invasive procedures.

Treatment
- Treatment depends on organism susceptibility and usually lasts for about 2–6 weeks.
- Initial blind therapy with flucloxacillin (or benzylpenicillin) + gentamicin.
- If penicillin allergic, have a prosthetic valve or methicillin-resistant *Staphylococcus aureus* (MRSA) suspected, substitute flucloxacillin (or benzylpenicillin) with vancomycin + rifampicin.
- Typical regimens are:
  - Streptococcal endocarditis: give IV benzylpenicillin + IV gentamicin.
  - Staphylococcal endocarditis: give IV flucloxacillin (or vancomycin + rifampicin if penicillin allergic or MRSA).
  - Enterococcal endocarditis: give IV amoxicillin (or vancomycin if penicillin allergic) + IV gentamicin.
  - For HACEK organisms (**H**aemophilus (*H. parainfluenzae*, *H. aphrophilus*, *H. paraphrophilus*), **A**ctinobacillus *actinomycetemcomitans* (*Aggregatibacter actinomycetemcomitans*) **C**ardiobacterium hominis, **E**ikenella corrodens, **K**ingella kingae) give IV amoxicillin + gentamicin. For fungal endocarditis the following are used depending on the specific organism: flucytosine, fluconazole, amphotericin.

- Consider surgery (valve replacement) if there is no response to antimicrobials, presence of heart failure, repeated embolic events, fungal endocarditis or myocardial abscess.

MALARIA

- Any patient with symptoms suggestive of infection, who has visited or been resident in areas where malaria is endemic, should be screened for malaria.
- Once diagnosed, treatment should be commenced.
- If species is not known, or the infection is mixed, initial treatment should be as for falciparum malaria with quinine, Malarone® (proguanil + atovaquone) or Riamet® (artemether + lumefantrine).
- Give IV quinine in those seriously ill or unable to swallow tablets. In cases of quinine resistance or not improving on quinine, IV artesunate can be used.
- If quinine is used also need to treat with doxycycline, clindamycin or Fansidar® together with, or after, a course of quinine.
- Benign malarias caused by *Plasmodium vivax*, *P. ovale* and *P. malariae* are treated with chloroquine.
- In cases of *P. vivax* and *P. ovale*, to prevent relapse parasites in the liver must be destroyed with primaquine after a course of chloroquine.
- In pregnancy, falciparum malaria is treated with quinine and clindamycin given with or after quinine; benign malarias are treated with chloroquine and primaquine used after delivery if required.
- Doxycycline, Fansidar®, Malarone® and Riamet® are best avoided in pregnancy.

MENINGITIS
Bacterial meningitis
Neonates
- Most likely organisms are:
    - Group B streptococci – treat with IV benzylpenicillin.
    - *Escherichia coli* – treat with IV cefotaxime.
    - *Listeria monocytogenes* – treat with IV amoxicillin + IV gentamicin.
- Blind therapy – IV benzylpenicillin + IV gentamicin.

Infant/toddler
- Most likely organisms are:
    - *Neisseria meningitidis* – treat with IV cefotaxime.
    - *Streptococcus pneumoniae* – treat with IV cefotaxime.
    - *Haemophilus influenzae* – treat with IV cefotaxime (incidence decreasing due to *H. influenzae* type b [Hib] vaccine).
- Blind therapy – IV cefotaxime.

From 4 years onwards
- Most likely organisms are:
    - *Neisseria meningitidis* – treat with IV cefotaxime.
    - *Streptococcus pneumoniae* – treat with IV cefotaxime.
- Blind therapy – IV cefotaxime.

Note
- IV fluids may be given if required.
- Dexamethasone should be given to decrease the risk of complications of meningitis (e.g. deafness, cerebral oedema) before, or with first dose of, antibiotic.
- Oral rifampicin is given to close contacts such as family members for a period of 48 hours to prevent spread of meningitis caused by *Neisseria meningitidis* or *Haemophilus influenzae*.
- Meningococcal meningitis is not to be confused with meningococcal septicaemia. Both are medical emergencies. If suspected, IV cefotaxime (or IM benzylpenicillin if in the community) should be given immediately *before* any investigations are undertaken.

Viral meningitis
- Viruses cause 'aseptic' meningitis, as opposed to the 'pyogenic' meningitis caused by bacteria such as *Neisseria meningitidis*. Causative agents of viral meningitis include mumps, herpes and enteroviruses.
- Treatment is supportive (e.g. bed rest, analgesia) as viral meningitis is self-limiting.

MUSCULOSKELETAL INFECTION
Septic arthritis
- After sending synovial fluid and blood cultures, start empirical antibiotics until sensitivities are known.
- Benzylpenicillin + flucloxacillin are used in combination empirically.
- Usual to treat with IV antibiotics for 2 weeks and continue with oral antibiotics for 4 weeks (discuss with microbiologist and orthopaedic team).
- Consider joint aspiration, lavage or debridement, especially if there is a prosthetic joint involved.

OTITIS MEDIA
- Otitis media is caused by bacteria or viruses. Common bacterial organisms are *Streptococcus pneumoniae* and *Haemophilus influenzae*.
- Most cases of acute otitis media are self-resolving, but consider antibiotics if no improvement after 72 hours. Oral co-amoxiclav or amoxicillin (or erythromycin in penicillin allergy) can be given (in severe cases given IV).
- In chronic otitis media consider myringotomy and grommet insertion.

RESPIRATORY TRACT INFECTIONS
Infective exacerbation of asthma/COPD
- Amoxicillin (or erythromycin or doxycycline in penicillin allergy).

Pneumonia
Community-acquired pneumonia
- Mostly caused by *Streptococcus pneumoniae*, followed by *Mycoplasma pneumoniae*.
- Treat with amoxicillin (plus erythromycin in severe cases).

Hospital-acquired pneumonia
*   Often caused by *Pseudomonas aeruginosa, Klebsiella pneumoniae, Staphylococcus aureus, Escherichia coli.*
*   Treatment is usually a broad-spectrum cephalosporin such as ceftazidime (plus an aminoglycoside in severe cases).

Atypical pneumonia
*   Mostly caused by *Mycoplasma pneumoniae, Chlamydia* spp., *Coxiella burnetii* and *Legionella* spp. infections.
*   Treat with erythromycin or tetracycline.

Tonsillitis/throat infections
*   More than half of tonsillitis cases are due to viral infection and therefore not amenable to antibiotic treatment. If you do decide to give an antibiotic, penicillin is the agent of choice, since the most common bacterial cause is *Streptococcus pyogenes.*
*   One of the aims of treating tonsillitis is to prevent rheumatic fever.
*   Remember that amoxicillin causes a rash if given to patients with infectious mononucleosis (i.e. EBV infection).

Tuberculosis
*   Phase 1: rifampicin + isoniazid + pyrazinamide for 2 months.
*   Phase 2: rifampicin + isoniazid for 4 months.
*   In cases of suspected isoniazid resistance, ethambutol may be given.
*   Give pyridoxine (vitamin B_6) throughout treatment as isoniazid can cause vitamin B_6 deficiency.

SEPTICAEMIA
*   Rehydrate.
*   Take cultures before starting antibiotic therapy, e.g. blood, urine, stool, sputum.
*   Need to cover Gram-positive, Gram-negative, anaerobic and possibly MRSA until septic foci found. Common regimes are IV amoxicillin + gentamicin with the addition of metronidazole if there are abdominal signs and vancomycin if MRSA is suspected.
*   When laboratory results are available, adapt antibiotic therapy if necessary.
*   Inotropes (e.g. norepinephrine) may be required if haemodynamically compromised despite IV fluids.

SEXUALLY TRANSMITTED DISEASES
*   Commonest cause is *Chlamydia trachomatis* followed by *Neisseria gonorrhoeae.*
*   Treat genital gonorrhoea with a single dose of cefixime or ciprofloxacin.
*   Treat genital chlamydial infection, non-gonococcal urethritis and non-specific genital infection with a single dose of azithromycin or a week's course of doxycycline to prevent complications such as infertility and ectopic pregnancies.
*   Remove intrauterine contraceptive device (IUCD) if present.

- Recommend barrier contraception or abstinence until recovery is made, to prevent spread of the infection.
- Contact screening is recommended.

SKIN INFECTIONS
Cellulitis
- Cellulitis is usually caused by a combination of staphylococci and Group A streptococci.
- Treat systemically with co-amoxiclav to cover both above-mentioned organisms or give flucloxacillin and benzylpenicillin in combination (or erythromycin if penicillin allergic).
- Depending on the site (e.g. diabetic foot infection), broad-spectrum cover may be required (e.g. gentamicin with co-amoxiclav).

Erysipelas
- Erysipelas is usually caused by Group A streptococci.
- Treat orally or IV depending on severity of infection with penicillin (or erythromycin if penicillin allergic).

Impetigo
- Impetigo is usually caused by staphylococci and Group A streptococci.
- For limited skin involvement, give topical fusidic acid (or mupirocin if MRSA).
- For more extensive skin involvement, give oral flucloxacillin or erythromycin.

Necrotizing fasciitis
- Causative agents are usually multiple, including Group A streptococci. Anaerobes are frequently involved due to the hypoxic tissue damage that occurs.
- Broad-spectrum antibiotics are the key. Treat systemically with penicillin and clindamycin, and add gentamicin if polymicrobial. Alternatively, give gentamicin and co-amoxiclav.
- Surgical debridement is usually required.
- Hyperbaric oxygen may be useful.

Animal and human bites
- Co-amoxiclav alone or doxycycline + metronidazole if penicillin allergic.
- Consider giving prophylactic treatment for tetanus, rabies and blood-borne viruses e.g. hepatitis B, HIV if clinically relevant.

URINARY TRACT INFECTIONS (UTIs)
Children
- Management should be initiated in consultation with a paediatrician.
- The child should be investigated for any underlying structural abnormalities (e.g. ureteric obstruction) and vesicoureteric reflux, while maintaining therapy with oral trimethoprim.

Adults
- Pyelonephritis – IV amoxicillin + gentamicin.
- Cystitis – oral trimethoprim (if pregnant, give oral amoxicillin or nitrofurantoin).

Note
- Cystitis is the most common form of UTI and can usually be treated with a single dose or a short course of antibiotic.
- Males who present with a first episode of cystitis or pyelonephritis should be investigated for underlying pathology (e.g. obstruction due to prostate enlargement or renal calculi).

Types of antibiotics

ANTIBACTERIALS

- Antibacterial agents work by acting on microbial components that are either absent or radically different in human cells (i.e. selective toxicity). There are three main mechanisms by which they arrest microbial growth, as detailed below.

Inhibition of cell wall synthesis
- *Penicillins:*
  - Benzylpenicillin (penicillin G), phenoxymethylpenicillin (penicillin V).
  - Broad-spectrum penicillins: amoxicillin, ampicillin.
  - Antipseudomonal penicillins: azlocillin, piperacillin, ticarcillin.
  - Beta-lactamase-resistant penicillins: cloxacillin, dicloxacillin, flucloxacillin.
- *Mecillinams:*
  - Pivmecillinam.
- *Cephalosporins:*
  - First-generation: cefazolin, cefradine, cefaclor, cefadroxil, cephalexin.
  - Second-generation: cefuroxime, cefamandole.
  - Third-generation: cefodizime, cefotaxime, ceftazidime, ceftizoxime, ceftriaxone, cefixime, ceftibuten, cefpodoxime proxetil.
  - Fourth-generation: cefepime, cefpirome.
  - Antipseudomonal cephalosporins: cefepime, ceftazidime.
- *Glycopeptides:*
  - Teicoplanin, vancomycin.
- *Carbapenems:*
  - Ertapenem, imipenem, meropenem.
- *Monobactams:*
  - Aztreonam.

Inhibition of nucleic acid synthesis
- *Quinolones:*
  - Ciprofloxacin, levofloxacin, nalidixic acid, norfloxacin, ofloxacin.
- *Trimethoprim.*
- *Sulfonamides:*
  - Sulfamethoxazole.
- *Nitroimidazoles:*
  - Metronidazole, ornidazole, tinidazole.
- *Nitrofurantoin.*
- *Rifampicin.*

Inhibition of protein synthesis
By acting on the 30S bacterial ribosomal subunit
- *Aminoglycosides:*
  - Amikacin, gentamicin, neomycin, streptomycin, tobramycin.

- *Tetracyclines***:**
  - Doxycycline, lymecycline, minocycline, oxytetracycline, tetracycline.

By acting on the 50S bacterial ribosomal subunit

- *Macrolides:*
  - Azithromycin, clarithromycin, erythromycin.
- *Linezolid.*
- *Clindamycin.*
- *Chloramphenicol.*
- *Fusidic acid.*

Treatments of choice

- Some common pathogens and antibiotics that can be used to treat them are shown below. It should be noted that resistance to many antibiotics is emerging and the regimens shown here are subject to change. Antibiotic guidelines vary between UK hospitals.

Pathogen	Treatment of choice
Anaerobes	Metronidazole
Bordetella pertussis	Erythromycin
Campylobacter spp.	Ciprofloxacin or erythromycin
Chlamydia trachomatis	Doxycycline
Clostridium difficile	Stop any antibiotics ± give oral metronidazole or oral vancomycin
Corynebacterium diphtheriae	Erythromycin
Enterococcus spp.	Amoxicillin/ ampicillin ± gentamicin
Escherichia coli	Trimethoprim for cystitis
	Ceftriaxone/gentamicin for serious infections
Giardia lamblia	Metronidazole
Haemophilus influenzae	Cefotaxime or co-amoxiclav
Legionella pneumophila	Erythromycin
Listeria monocytogenes	Ampicillin + gentamicin
Mycobacterium tuberculosis	Rifampicin + isoniazid + pyrazinamide (± ethambutol)
Mycoplasma pneumoniae	Erythromycin or tetracycline
Neisseria gonorrhoea	Cefixime or ciprofloxacin
Neisseria meningitidis	Any beta-lactam (ceftriaxone, cefotaxime)
Pseudomonas aeruginosa	Aminoglycoside + antipseudomonal penicillin
Salmonella spp.	Ciprofloxacin
Shigella dysenteriae	Ciprofloxacin
Staphylococcus spp.	Flucloxacillin if not methicillin-resistant, vancomycin for MRSA
Streptococcus spp.	Penicillin or cephalosporin
Vibrio cholerae	Tetracycline

ANTIFUNGALS

- Fungal infections (termed mycoses) are difficult to treat. Being eukaryotic, their metabolic pathways are more similar to mammalian cells and therefore present fewer targets for chemotherapy. They usually involve the skin, nails or mucous membranes. Systemic fungal infections usually occur in immunocompromised individuals. There are four main classes of antifungal drugs:

  1. *Imidazoles.* These act by inhibiting synthesis of lipids in the fungal cell membrane (e.g. clotrimazole, miconazole, ketoconazole).

  2. *Polyenes.* These act by forming pores in the fungal membrane, leading to cell death (e.g. amphotericin, nystatin).

  3. *Triazoles.* These act by a mechanism similar to the imidazoles (e.g. fluconazole, itraconazole).

  4. *Others.* These include flucytosine, griseofulvin and terbinafine.

Treatments of choice

Fungus	Treatment of choice
Aspergillus spp.	Amphotericin
Blastomyces spp.	Itraconazole
Candida spp.	Local therapy: nystatin/clotrimazole
	Systemic therapy: fluconazole/amphotericin
Coccidioides spp.	Amphotericin
Cryptococcus neoformans	Amphotericin/fluconazole
Histoplasma capsulatum	Amphotericin/itraconazole
Malassezia furfur (*Pityriasis versicolor*)	Local therapy: terbinafine
	Systemic therapy: itraconazole
Paracoccidioides spp.	Itraconazole
Dermatophytes (*Epidermophyton* spp., *Microsporum* spp., *Trichophyton* spp.)	Griseofulvin/imidazoles

ANTIVIRALS

- Viruses, which live and replicate inside human cells, make use of the metabolic pathways of the host cell. It is thus very difficult to direct treatment selectively against the virus without in some way adversely affecting the patient.
- There are three general mechanisms by which antiviral agents work:

  1. Inhibition of viral nucleic acid synthesis (e.g. aciclovir, foscarnet, ganciclovir, ribavirin, zidovudine).

2. Immunomodulatory action (e.g. immunoglobulins [Ig], interferons).

3. Inhibition of specific viral targets (e.g. amantadine, oseltamivir, pleconaril, ritonavir, zanamivir).

Treatments of choice

Virus	Treatment of choice
CMV	Ganciclovir
Hepatitis B	Peginterferon or nucleotide or nucleoside
Hepatitis C	Peginterferon and ribavirin
Hepatitis D	Treat hepatitis B
Herpes simplex	Aciclovir
HIV	Highly active antiretroviral therapy (HAART) (see pp. 154–155)
Influenza A	Oseltamivir/zanamivir
Respiratory syncitial virus	Consider nebulized ribavirin
Varicella zoster	Aciclovir, valaciclovir

Drugs

ACICLOVIR

Class: Antiviral agent

Indications
* Infections caused by alpha herpes viruses (herpes simplex types 1 and 2, varicella zoster virus).

Mechanism of action
* Aciclovir is selectively taken up by virus-infected cells. It is preferentially phosphorylated by herpes virus-encoded thymidine kinase to aciclovir monophosphate. This is then converted to aciclovir triphosphate by cellular phosphokinases. Aciclovir triphosphate is incorporated into herpes DNA and acts as a chain terminator.

Adverse effects
* *Rare*: rash (topical lotion); nausea, vomiting, headache (oral route); renal impairment (if given too quickly IV); confusion, hallucinations (IV route); inflammation at the drip site (if there is leakage into tissues).

Contraindications
* None.
* Caution:
  * Pregnancy and breastfeeding.

Interactions
* *Probenecid*: increases the plasma concentration of aciclovir by decreasing its excretion (this does not apply to topical aciclovir preparations).

Route of administration
* Oral, topical, IV.

Note
* Aciclovir is prescribed for herpes simplex types 1 and 2 infections (genital herpes, cold sores, encephalitis, eye infections). It is also used to treat shingles and chickenpox, both caused by varicella zoster virus.
* Famciclovir and valaciclovir are alternatives to aciclovir that may be used in the treatment of herpes simplex and zoster infections.
* If encephalitis is suspected, IV aciclovir should be given immediately.
* In aciclovir resistance, foscarnet or cidofovir should be used.
* Valganciclovir is used as an oral preparation to treat CMV infections in those who are immunocompromised but in severe infection cidofovir, foscarnet or ganciclovir are used intravenously.

Related drugs
* Famciclovir, valaciclovir.

AMOXICILLIN

Class: Beta-lactam antibiotic

Indications
* Wide range of infections caused by Gram-positive (e.g. *Streptococcus* spp., *Staphylococcus* spp.) and Gram-negative (e.g. *Haemophilus influenzae*) bacteria.
* Part of *Helicobacter pylori* eradication therapy.

Mechanism of action
* Amoxicillin is a broad-spectrum bactericidal antibiotic.
* It inhibits bacterial cell wall synthesis by preventing formation of cross-links between peptidoglycan chains that constitute the bacterial cell wall.

Adverse effects
* *Common*: rash, diarrhoea, nausea, vomiting, candida vaginitis.
* *Rare*: anaphylaxis, antibiotic-associated colitis, blood disorders.

Contraindications
* Penicillin hypersensitivity.

Interactions
* *COC pill*: amoxicillin may reduce the effectiveness of the pill.
* *Probenecid*: decreases excretion of amoxicillin.

Route of administration
* Oral, IM, IV.

Note
* Certain strains of bacteria produce the enzyme beta-lactamase, which inactivates amoxicillin. In order to prevent this inactivation, amoxicillin can be usefully combined with clavulanic acid (known as co-amoxiclav).
* Amoxicillin characteristically causes a rash if given to patients with infectious mononucleosis.
* Patients also taking the COC pill should be advised to take other contraceptive precautions during and for 7 days after treatment e.g. condoms.

Related drugs
* Ampicillin (reduced oral bioavailability compared to amoxycillin).

BENZYLPENICILLIN (PENICILLIN G)

Class: Beta-lactam antibiotic

Indications
*   Infections caused by *Streptococcus* spp.,*Neisseria meningitidis* and *N. gonorrhoeae*.
*   Also used in infections caused by *Treponema pallidum*, *Corynebacterium diphtheriae*, *Clostridium tetani*, *Bacillus anthracis*, *Leptospira* spp. and other susceptible organisms.

Mechanism of action
*   Benzylpenicillin is a bactericidal antibiotic.
*   It inhibits bacterial cell wall synthesis by preventing formation of cross-links between peptidoglycan chains that constitute the bacterial cell wall.

Adverse effects
*   *Common*: rash, diarrhoea.
*   *Rare*: anaphylaxis; bone marrow suppression and convulsions in high doses, renal impairment.

Contraindications
*   Penicillin hypersensitivity.

Interactions
*   *Probenecid*: decreases excretion of benzylpenicillin (a useful interaction that allows dose reduction of penicillin).

Route of administration
*   IV, IM.

Note
*   Benzylpenicillin is inactivated by the enzyme beta-lactamase, which is produced by many organisms (e.g. most *Staphylococcus* spp., some strains of *Escherichia coli* and *Pseudomonas* spp.). These organisms can be treated with beta-lactamase-resistant penicillins or antipseudomonal penicillins.
*   In cases of penicillin allergy, erythromycin can be given.
*   A total of 1–10% of patients given a penicillin experience an allergic reaction. Less than 0.05% suffer an anaphylaxis. These hypersensitivity reactions are triggered by the breakdown products of penicillin.

Related drugs
*   Penicillin V (oral equivalent of benzylpenicillin).

CEFUROXIME

Class: Second-generation cephalosporin (beta-lactam antibiotic)

Indications
* Infections caused by Gram-positive (e.g. *Streptococcus* spp., *Staphylococcus* spp.) and Gram-negative bacteria (e.g. *Escherichia coli*, *Haemophilus influenzae*).

Mechanism of action
* Cefuroxime inhibits bacterial cell wall synthesis by preventing formation of cross-links between peptidoglycan chains that constitute the bacterial cell wall.

Adverse effects
* *Common*: nausea, vomiting, diarrhoea.
* *Rare*: interstitial nephritis, hepatic impairment, blood disorders, rash, neurological symptoms, antibiotic-associated colitis.

Contraindications
* Acute porphyria.
* Caution:
    * Penicillin allergy (see below).

Interactions
* *Probenecid*: increases the plasma concentration of cefuroxime by decreasing its excretion.
* *Warfarin*: cefuroxime may enhance the anticoagulant effect of warfarin.

Route of administration
* Oral, IM, IV, eye drops.

Note
* Clinically, cephalosporins are commonly used to treat septicaemia, meningitis, pneumonia, UTIs and peritonitis.
* Currently there are four generations of cephalosporins available (see p. 161).
* First- and second-generation cephalosporins are used against both Gram-negative and Gram-positive organisms.
* Third-generation cephalosporins are less toxic, more efficacious and more specific towards Gram-negative organisms.
* Fourth-generation cephalosporins have increased anti-staphylococcal activity and are more active against Enterobacteriaceae than third-generation cephalosporins.
* About 10% of patients who are allergic to penicillin will have an allergic reaction to cephalosporins. This is due to a similar chemical structure.

CHLORAMPHENICOL

Class: Antibacterial agent

Indications
* Gram-positive and Gram-negative bacterial infections, including anaerobes.
* *Rickettsia* spp., *Mycoplasma* spp. and *Chlamydia* spp. infections.

Mechanism of action
* Chloramphenicol is a bacteriostatic antibiotic.
* It binds to the 50S subunit of the bacterial ribosome and thereby inhibits protein synthesis. This prevents bacterial reproduction.

Adverse effects
* *Common*: nausea, diarrhoea, anorexia.
* *Rare*: reversible or irreversible aplastic anaemia, optic and peripheral neuritis, grey baby syndrome in neonates, urticaria.

Contraindications
* Pregnancy.
* Breastfeeding.
* Acute porphyria.

Interactions
* *Phenytoin:* concomittant use increase the risk of phenytoin toxicity.
* *Warfarin*: concomitant use increases the anticoagulant increased effect of warfarin.

Route of administration
* Oral, IV, topical.

Note
* Clinically chloramphenicol is used in otitis externa and conjunctivitis topically. It is also used in bacterial meningitis in those allergic to penicillin or cephalosporins.
* Chloramphenicol is a potent broad-spectrum antibiotic that should only be used second line, owing to its potentially lethal adverse effects (aplastic anaemia).
* Aplastic anaemia may occur during or after chloramphenicol treatment. If occurring after, it is usually irreversible.
* Patients should not receive any vaccinations while on chloramphenicol treatment as their effect is reduced.

CIPROFLOXACIN

Class: Quinolone antibiotic

Indications
• Mainly Gram-negative infections (e.g. *Salmonella* spp., *Pseudomonas* spp., *Campylobacter* spp., *Neisseria* spp., *Escherichia coli, Haemophilus influenzae*).
• Some Gram-positive infections (e.g. *Streptococcus pneumoniae, Enterococcus faecalis*).

Mechanism of action
• Ciprofloxacin is a broad-spectrum bactericidal antibiotic.
• It inhibits the activity of the bacterial enzyme DNA gyrase, which is necessary for coiling and replication of bacterial DNA. Human cells do not contain DNA gyrase.

Adverse effects
• *Common*: nausea, vomiting, abdominal pain, diarrhoea.
• *Rare*: insomnia, confusion, convulsions, hepatitis, tendon damage/rupture, photosensitivity.

Contraindications
• None.
• Caution:
    • Epilepsy (ciprofloxacin lowers the seizure threshold).
    • Pregnancy.
    • Breastfeeding.
    • Children (animal studies have shown damage to cartilage).

Interactions
• *Ciclosporin*: concomitant use of ciprofloxacin and ciclosporin increases the risk of nephrotoxicity.
• *Theophylline*: ciprofloxacin may increase the risk of convulsions.
• *Warfarin*: ciprofloxacin enhances the anticoagulant effect of warfarin.

Route of administration
• Oral, IV, eye drops.

Note
• Clinically ciprofloxacin is used in respiratory tract, GI tract and complicated UTIs. It is also used in gonorrhoea and in anthrax infections.
• Ciprofloxacin is mainly used to treat bacterial infections that are resistant to other commonly used antibiotics. Bacteria may become resistant to quinolones, owing to a mutation in their DNA gyrase. There is now a high incidence of resistant staphylococci.
• The risk of tendon damage by quinolones is further increased with concomitant use of corticosteroids.

Related drugs
• Levofloxacin, nalidixic acid, norfloxacin, ofloxacin.

CLOTRIMAZOLE

Class: Imidazole antifungal

Indications
• Superficial, vaginal and mucous membrane fungal infections.

Mechanism of action
• Clotrimazole is a broad-spectrum antifungal agent.
• It inhibits production of ergosterol (a steroid) in the fungal cell wall. This renders the cell wall unstable with ensuing efflux of phosphorus compounds, which in turn leads to breakdown of nucleic acids in the cell and potassium efflux. These actions result in fungal cell death.

Adverse effects
• *Rare*: dyspareunia (with vaginal application), GI symptoms, itching, rash, reversible hepatic impairment.

Contraindications
• First trimester of pregnancy.

Interactions
• *Tacrolimus*: concomitant use may result in an increased plasma concentration of tacrolimus.

Route of administration
• Topical, vaginal, oral.

Note
• Clinically, clotrimazole is used in dermatophyte, yeast and *Malassezia furfur* infections.
• Triazole antifungals, such as itraconazole, are more specific towards fungal enzymes than imidazoles. This results in fewer adverse effects.
• Clotrimazole should not be applied in proximity of the eyes.

Related drugs
• Other topical antifungal drugs: econazole, ketoconazole, miconazole, nystatin, sulconazole, tioconazole.

ERYTHROMYCIN

Class: Macrolide antibiotic

Indications

*   Alternative to penicillin in penicillin allergy.
*   Infections caused by Gram-positive (e.g. *Corynebacterium diphtheriae*) and some Gram-negative bacteria (e.g. *Bordetella pertussis*).
*   *Mycoplasma pneumoniae*, *Legionella pneumophila*, *Treponema pallidum* and *Chlamydia* spp. infections.
*   Acne.
*   Rosacea.

Mechanism of action

*   Erythromycin is a broad-spectrum bacteriostatic antibiotic.
*   It inhibits bacterial protein synthesis by reversibly binding to the 50S subunit of the bacterial ribosome.

Adverse effects

*   *Common*: nausea, vomiting, abdominal pain, diarrhoea, rash, phlebitis (when injected into a peripheral vein).
*   *Rare*: reversible hearing loss (with high doses); cholestatic jaundice (with therapy lasting longer than 2 weeks), pseudomembranous colitis.

Contraindications

*   None.
*   Caution:
    *   Liver disease.
    *   Renal impairment.
    *   Pregnancy.
    *   Breastfeeding.

Interactions

*   *Ciclosporin*: erythromycin increases the plasma concentration of ciclosporin.
*   *Digoxin*: effects of digoxin are enhanced by erythromycin.
*   *Theophylline*: erythromycin increases the plasma concentration of theophylline.
*   *Warfarin*: erythromycin enhances the anticoagulant effect of warfarin.
*   *Note*: erythromycin inhibits hepatic drug-metabolizing enzymes; hence a wide range of further interactions exists.

Route of administration

*   Oral, IV.

Note

*   A course of erythromycin of longer than 14 days increases the risk of hepatic damage.
*   Azithromycin and clarithromycin cause fewer GI side-effects than erythromycin.
*   Macrolides are the treatment of choice in *Legionella*, *Mycoplasma* and *Campylobacter* infections.
*   Azithromycin is used as single dose therapy in the treatment of sexually transmitted diseases, i.e. genital chlamydial, non-gonococcal urethritis.

Related drugs

*   Azithromycin, clarithromycin, spiramycin, telithromycin.

FLUCLOXACILLIN

Class: Beta-lactam antibiotic

Indications
*   Beta-lactam-resistant *Staphylococcus* spp. infections (e.g. otitis externa, cellulitis).

Mechanism of action
*   Flucloxacillin is a narrow-spectrum bactericidal antibiotic.
*   It inhibits bacterial cell wall synthesis by preventing cross-linking between peptidoglycan chains that constitute the bacterial cell wall.

Adverse effects
*   *Common*: hypersensitivity (rash, urticaria, fever, joint pains).
*   *Rare*: anaphylaxis, cholestatic jaundice, hepatitis.

Contraindications
*   Penicillin hypersensitivity.

Interactions
*   *COC pill*: flucloxacillin can reduce the contraceptive effect by interfering with gut flora.

Route of administration
*   Oral, IM, IV.

Note
*   Unlike other penicillins, flucloxacillin is resistant to staphylococcal beta-lactamase. This bacterial enzyme cleaves the beta-lactam ring of certain penicillins by hydrolysis, rendering them inactive.
*   Flucloxacillin-resistant strains of *Staphylococcus aureus* (i.e. MRSA) have emerged in many hospitals. Therapy with vancomycin or teicoplanin is usually indicated for these organisms.
*   Patients taking both the COC pill and flucloxacillin must be informed of the reduced contraceptive effect.
*   The risk of cholestatic jaundice is increased if flucloxacillin is given for longer than 2 weeks.

GENTAMICIN

Class: Aminoglycoside antibiotic

Indications
* Serious infections caused by aerobic Gram-negative bacteria, e.g. septicaemia, pyelonephritis, hospital-acquired pneumonia and biliary tract infections.

Mechanism of action
* Gentamicin is bactericidal.
* Gentamicin inhibits bacterial protein synthesis by binding irreversibly to the 30S subunit of the bacterial ribosome.

Adverse effects
* *Rare*: nephrotoxicity, ototoxicity (gentamicin can damage the 8th cranial nerve), hypomagnesaemia.

Contraindications
* Myasthenia gravis.
* Caution:
    * Pregnancy (gentamicin crosses the placenta and can damage the fetal 8th cranial nerve).
    * Renal impairment (use lower dose).

Interactions
* *Ciclosporin*: potentiates nephrotoxic effect of gentamicin.
* *Cytotoxics*: potentiate nephrotoxic effect of gentamicin.
* *Loop diuretics*: potentiate ototoxic effect of gentamicin.
* *Neostigmine, pyridostigmine*: gentamicin antagonizes the effects of these drugs.

Route of administration
* IV, IM, topical (eye drops), intrathecal.

Note
* Gentamicin has a narrow therapeutic window, therefore therapeutic drug monitoring is essential. Either given as a once daily or multiple daily dose regime.
* Gentamicin is usually combined with penicillin and/or metronidazole in blind therapy for serious infections.
* Amikacin can be used to treat serious infections caused by Gram-negative bacilli that are resistant to gentamicin.
* Tobramycin is administered by nebulizer to treat chronic *Pseudomonas aeruginosa* infections in patients with cystic fibrosis.
* Streptomycin is only used in the treatment of tuberculosis.
* Aminoglycosides can precipitate a myasthenic crisis.

Related drugs
* Amikacin, neomycin, streptomycin, tobramycin.

METRONIDAZOLE

Class: Nitroimidazole antibiotic

Indications
* Anaerobic and protozoan infections.
* Part of *Helicobacter pylori* eradication therapy.
* Rosacea.
* Pseudomembranous colitis.

Mechanism of action
* Metronidazole is a bacteriostatic antibiotic.
* It is broken down into toxic compounds (free radicals) within microbes that possess anaerobic or microaerophilic metabolism. These toxic compounds arrest growth by interfering with their nucleic acid function and synthesis.

Adverse effects
* *Common*: nausea, vomiting, anorexia, diarrhoea, metallic taste in mouth.
* *Rare*: anaphylaxis, drowsiness, headache, hepatitis, blood disorders, peripheral neuropathy with long-term use.

Contraindications
* None.
* Caution:
    * Pregnancy and breastfeeding.
    * Hepatic impairment.

Interactions
* *Alcohol*: this causes a disulfiram-like reaction with metronidazole (see below).
* *Phenytoin*: metronidazole increases the plasma concentration of phenytoin by inhibiting its metabolism.
* *Warfarin*: metronidazole enhances the anticoagulant effect of warfarin by inhibiting its metabolism.

Route of administration
* Oral, IV, rectal.

Note
* Important to warn patients about stopping treatment if they experience symptoms of peripheral neuropathy in the limbs.
* Metronidazole is commonly used to treat dental infections as these are mostly caused by anaerobes. It is also widely used as prophylaxis and treatment of intra-abdominal infections.
* Patients should be warned of the disulfiram-like reaction that occurs if alcohol is taken while on metronidazole treatment (flushing, abdominal pain, hypotension). This reaction can occur up to 3 days after stopping treatment.
* Tinidazole is similar to metronidazole but has a longer duration of action.

Related drugs
* Tinidazole.

QUININE

Class: Antimalarial

Indications
- Treatment of malaria caused by *Plasmodium falciparum*.

Mechanism of action
- Quinine is toxic to the malaria parasite, specifically by interfering with the parasite's ability to break down and digest haemoglobin, thus starving the parasite and/or causing the build-up of toxic levels of partially degraded haemoglobin in the parasite.

Adverse effects
- *Common*: tinnitus, poor hearing, nausea, vomiting.
- *Rare*: arrhythmias, visual disturbances, hypoglycaemia, renal impairment, blood disorders.

Contraindications
- Myasthenia gravis.
- Optic neuritis.
- Tinnitus.
- Haemoglobinuria.

Interactions
- *Amiodarone, flecainide, terfenadine:* increased risk of dysrhythmias.
- *Digoxin:* quinine increases the concentration of digoxin.

Route of administration
- Oral, IV.

Note
- Quinine is also used for the treatment of malaria when the infective species is not known or in mixed infection.
- If seriously ill, give quinine IV and switch to oral preparation once patient starts to improve.
- Quinine may precipitate haemolysis in those with glucose-6-phosphate dehydrogenase (G6PD) deficiency.
- If quinine is used in the treatment of malaria also need to treat with doxycycline, clindamycin or Fansidar® together with or after a course of quinine.

RIFAMPICIN

Class: Antituberculous agent

Indications
- Tuberculosis.
- Leprosy.
- Prophylaxis of meningococcal meningitis and Hib infection in contacts of cases.

Mechanism of action
- Rifampicin inhibits the DNA-dependent RNA polymerase isoenzyme in bacteria (but not in human cells) and is thus bactericidal.

Adverse effects
- *Common*: disturbance of LFTs; orange-coloured tears, urine and sputum.
- *Rare*: hepatitis, rash, thrombocytopenia, nausea, vomiting, flu-like illness, orange discoloration of soft contact lenses.

Contraindications
- Jaundice.

Interactions
- *Calcium-channel blockers, corticosteroids and phenytoin*: rifampicin accelerates the metabolism of these drugs, thus reducing their effects.
- *Oestrogens and progestogens*: rifampicin accelerates the metabolism of the COC pill, thus reducing the contraceptive effect.
- *Warfarin*: rifampicin increases the metabolism of warfarin, thus decreasing its effect.
- *Note*: rifampicin induces hepatic drug-metabolising enzymes; hence a wide range of further interactions exists.

Route of administration
- Oral, IV.

Note
- Resistance to rifampicin can develop rapidly if it is used alone. Therefore it is usually given in combination with ethambutol, pyrazinamide and isoniazid in patients with tuberculosis.
- LFTs should be carried out before treatment. The patient should be advised how to recognize signs of liver dysfunction. If these occur, LFTs should be repeated.
- Compliance may be difficult, as treatment for tuberculosis lasts for 6–9 months.
- Rifampicin can also be used in the treatment of legionnaire's disease, endocarditis, brucellosis and other staphylococcal infections, in combination with other antimicrobials.
- Rifampicin can also be used to treat pruritus in primary biliary cirrhosis.

TETRACYCLINE

Class: Tetracycline antibiotic

Indications
- Infections caused by *Coxiella burnetii, Mycoplasma* spp., *Leptospira icterohaemorrhagiae, Chlamydia* spp., *Rickettsia* spp., *Borrelia burgdorferi* and other susceptible organisms.
- Acne.
- Rosacea.
- Part of *Helicobacter pylori* eradication therapy.

Mechanism of action
- Tetracycline is a broad-spectrum bacteriostatic antibiotic.
- It undergoes selective uptake into bacterial cells and binds reversibly to the 30S subunit of the ribosome. This disrupts protein synthesis by interfering with RNA translation.

Adverse effects
- *Common*: nausea, vomiting, diarrhoea.
- *Rare*: benign intracranial hypertension, photosensitivity, rash, blood disorders, hepatic impairment, dysphagia, pancreatitis, renal impairment.

Contraindications
- Children.
- Pregnancy.
- Breastfeeding.
- Renal impairment.
- SLE.

Interactions
- *Antacids*: decrease the absorption of tetracycline.
- *Ferrous sulphate*: tetracycline decreases the absorption of ferrous sulphate.

Route of administration
- Oral, topical, IM, IV.

Note
- Most Gram-positive and several Gram-negative bacteria are now resistant to tetracycline (resistance is mediated by plasmids).
- Tetracycline binds to calcium and is therefore deposited in growing bones and teeth. This leads to discoloration of teeth and should therefore not be given to children under 12 years of age or to lactating or pregnant women.
- Tetracycline should not be taken with food or milk (impaired absorption).
- Doxycycline is preferred to tetracycline as it does not affect renal function and its absorption is not decreased by milk. Also it can be used in the treatment of infective exacerbation of COPD as it has activity against *Haemophilus influenzae*.

Related drugs
- Doxycycline, lymecycline, minocycline, oxytetracycline.

TRIMETHOPRIM

Class: Antifolate antibiotic

Indications
- Treatment and prophylaxis of UTIs.
- Prostatitis.

Mechanism of action
- Trimethoprim reduces bacterial production of folate by inhibiting the bacterial enzyme dihydrofolate reductase. Trimethoprim has a 50 000 times greater affinity for bacterial dihydrofolate reductase than for human dihydrofolate reductase.
- Trimethoprim is bacteriostatic, as folate is an essential co-factor in DNA synthesis.

Adverse effects
- *Rare*: bone marrow suppression, nausea, vomiting, rash, toxic epidermal necrolysis, hyperkalaemia.

Contraindications
- Pregnancy (due to teratogenic risk).
- Blood disorders (e.g. anaemia, thrombocytopenia).

Interactions
- *Ciclosporin*: concomitant use of ciclosporin and trimethoprim increases the risk of nephrotoxicity.
- *Cytotoxics*: concomitant use increases the risk of bone marrow toxicity.
- *Pyrimethamine*: concomitant use of pyrimethamine and trimethoprim can enhance the antifolate effect.

Route of administration
- Oral.

Note
- Resistance to trimethoprim is common.
- Trimethoprim can be used in combination with sulfamethoxazole (a sulfonamide) as co-trimoxazole, which is bactericidal. This combination produces synergistic activity and is especially effective for *Pneumocystis jiroveci (P. carinii)* pneumonia.
- Co-trimoxazole is associated with serious adverse effects such as blood dyscrasias and Stevens–Johnson syndrome, hence its use is limited to treatment of toxoplasmosis, nocardiosis and only in respiratory infections and UTIs when there is good rationale for use.

VANCOMYCIN

Class: Glycopeptide antibiotic

Indications
- Infections caused by aerobic and anaerobic Gram-positive bacteria including MRSA.
- Pseudomembranous colitis (caused by *Clostridium difficile*).
- Treatment of peritonitis caused by peritoneal dialysis catheter.

Mechanism of action
- Vancomycin is a bactericidal antibiotic.
- It inhibits bacterial cell wall synthesis by binding to precursor units of the cell wall.
- Vancomycin also interferes with ribonucleic acid (RNA) synthesis and permeability of the bacterial cell wall.

Adverse effects
- *Common*: anorexia, nausea.
- *Rare*: agranulocytosis, 'red man' syndrome (flushing of the upper body), renal failure, hearing loss, rash, fever.

Contraindications
- Hypersensitivity.

Interactions
- *Ciclosporin*: the risk of nephrotoxicity is increased.
- *Loop diuretics*: the risk of ototoxicity is increased.
- *Oestrogens*: possible reduced contraceptive effect.

Route of administration
- Oral (for pseudomembranous colitis), IV, added to dialysis fluid via peritoneal catheter.

Note
- Clinically vancomycin is used in staphylococcal enterocolitis or other staphylococcal infections (e.g. endocarditis).
- Agranulocytosis can occur 1 or more weeks after starting IV vancomycin. It is often reversible by stopping vancomycin.
- Teicoplanin is similar to vancomycin and can be given by IM and IV injection and does not require drug monitoring.
- Vancomycin resistant enterococci (VRE) strains first emerged in 1987 and have spread rapidly since then. Prevention of VRE relies on good hygiene (e.g. hand washing) and careful, restricted use of vancomycin.
- Linezolid is an antibiotic that can be used when vancomycin is inappropriate to treat respiratory, skin or other infections caused by MRSA. This drug can cause blood disorders and optic neuropathy.

Related drugs
- Teicoplanin.

ZIDOVUDINE

Class: Nucleoside reverse transcriptase inhibitor (NRTI)

Indications
* Part of combination therapy for HIV infection.
* Prevention of HIV transmission from mother to fetus and in those exposed to HIV infected blood following needle-stick injury.

Mechanism of action
* Zidovudine is a nucleoside analogue. It is phosphorylated inside cells to form zidovudine triphosphate, which is a competitive inhibitor of viral reverse transcriptase. Zidovudine triphosphate is also incorporated into proviral DNA, thus terminating DNA chain elongation.
* *Note*: zidovudine does not eradicate HIV from the body.

Adverse effects
* *Common*: anaemia, neutropenia, headache, insomnia, nausea, abdominal pain, diarrhoea.
* *Rare*: pancreatitis, hepatic impairment, lactic acidosis, lipodystrophy syndrome (fat redistribution, dyslipidaemia, insulin resistance), osteonecrosis.

Contraindications
* Low neutrophil count.
* Severe anaemia.
* Breastfeeding.

Interactions
* *Ganciclovir*: severe myelosuppression if given with zidovudine.
* *Probenecid*: increases the risk of zidovudine toxicity by raising its plasma concentration.

Route of administration
* Oral, IV.

Note
* Treatment for HIV involves two NRTIs with either a non-NRTI or a protease inhibitor.
* Protease inhibitors have a similar side effect profile to NRTIs but also cause hyperglycaemia.
* Resistance to zidovudine develops as a result of mutations in viral reverse transcriptase. Combined therapy is given in order to prevent emergence of resistant strains (see p. 154).
* Therapy is guided by HIV viral load and CD4 count.

Related drugs
* Abacavir, didanosine, emtricitabine, lamivudine, stavudine, tenofovir.

IMMUNIZATION

Management guidelines (pp. 183–185)
Recommended immunization programme in the UK
Adult immunizations
Travel immunizations
Contraindications to all vaccines
Contraindications to live vaccines

Vaccines (pp. 186–196)
Bacillus Calmette–Guérin (BCG) vaccine
Diphtheria vaccine
Haemophilus influenzae type B (HIB) vaccine
Hepatitis B vaccine
Human papilloma virus (HPV) vaccine
Influenza vaccine
Meningococcal group C vaccine
Mumps measles rubella (MMR) vaccine
Pertussis vaccine
Poliomyelitis vaccine
Tetanus vaccine

Management guidelines

RECOMMENDED IMMUNIZATION PROGRAMME IN THE UK

Vaccine	Age
Hepatitis B (for neonates at risk)	Birth, 1 month and 6 months
Diphtheria, tetanus, pertussis (DTP), poliomyelitis, Hib – combined vaccine	2, 3 and 4 months
Pneumococcal and meningococcal	2, 4 months
Hib, meningococcal	12 months
MMR, pneumococcal	13 months
DTP, poliomyelitis, MMR	3–5 years (preschool booster)
HPV	Girls 12–13 years (3 doses within 6 months)
Diphtheria, tetanus (DT) (low dose), poliomyelitis	13–18 years (school-leavers)

The Hands–on Guide to Clinical Pharmacology, 3rd Edition. By S Chatu.
Published 2010 by Blackwell Publishing Ltd.

Note
*   If the immunization course is interrupted, there is no need to restart the entire course.
*   Jet guns should not be used for vaccination due to the risk of transmission of blood-borne infections.
*   Immunization schedules may differ between countries. National immunization guidelines should be consulted.
*   Most vaccines used for the primary course and boosters are combined products to prevent the number of injections administered.

ADULT IMMUNIZATIONS
*   Most vaccinations are given during childhood.
*   MMR vaccine:
    *   Women of childbearing age who have not received 2 doses in childhood, or are not positive for the rubella antibody, should be offered vaccination but pregnancy must be excluded before immunization.
*   DTP vaccines:
    *   If not previously immunized, 3 doses at 4-week intervals and booster dose 1 year later and again 5–10 years later.
*   In high-risk groups, the following vaccinations should be considered:
    *   BCG.
    *   Hepatitis B.
    *   Tetanus.
    *   Influenza.
    *   Pneumococcal.

TRAVEL IMMUNIZATIONS
*   Individuals should visit their GP well in advance of departure to obtain advice about which vaccines will be required for their trip.
*   Some vaccines need to be given several weeks before travel to provide adequate protection.
*   Travel vaccines include:
    *   Typhoid.
    *   Hepatitis A.
    *   Hepatitis B.
    *   Meningitis C.
    *   DTP (combined in one vaccine).
    *   Yellow fever, rabies.
    *   Japanese B encephalitis and tick-borne encephalitis.

CONTRAINDICATIONS TO ALL VACCINES
*   Acute febrile illness.
*   Severe reaction to a previous dose.

CONTRADICTIONS TO LIVE VACCINES (BCG, MMR, POLIOMYELITIS, YELLOW FEVER)
*   Acute febrile illness.
*   Severe reaction to a previous dose.

- Immunocompromised patients.
- Pregnancy.
- HIV (omit BCG, but MMR and inactivated poliomyelitis vaccine can be given).
- High-dose corticosteroids (wait for 3 months after stopping steroids).
- Receiving chemotherapy and/or radiotherapy (wait for 6 months after stopping therapy).
- Another live vaccine within the previous 3 weeks.
- Certain malignant conditions (e.g. leukaemia, malignancy of the reticuloendothelial system).

Vaccines

BACILLUS CALMETTE–GUÉRIN (BCG) VACCINE

Class: Live attenuated vaccine

Indications
- Prophylaxis of tuberculosis in high-risk individuals.
- Primary or recurrent carcinoma of the bladder.

Mechanism of action
- BCG vaccine contains a live attenuated strain derived from *Mycobacterium bovis*. This induces a hypersensitivity reaction and thereby stimulates cell-mediated immunity against *M. tuberculosis*.
- Instillation into the bladder results in chronic granulomatous cystitis, an immunological response thought to be essential for anti-tumour activity.

Adverse effects
- *Common*: ulcer at injection site.
- *Rare*: axillary lymphadenopathy, tuberculosis (in the immunocompromised); cystitis, haematuria, urinary frequency, systemic BCG infection (with bladder instillation).

Contraindications
- Acute febrile illness.
- Immunocompromised patients (e.g. steroid therapy, immunosuppressive drugs, HIV, malignancy).
- Pregnancy.
- Receiving chemotherapy and/or radiotherapy (defer BCG vaccine for 6 months).
- The first 3 weeks following another live vaccine.
- Malignant conditions of the reticuloendothelial system.
- Leukaemia.

Interactions
- None.

Route of administration
- Intradermal, topical.

Note
- BCG is given to healthcare workers and laboratory staff in the UK.
- Neonates and infants born in areas where tuberculosis is endemic should be vaccinated.
- BCG vaccine should only be given if the Heaf test or Mantoux test is negative (with exception of children under 6 years of age).
- An ulcer usually appears at the site of injection 2–3 weeks after the vaccination. This normally heals within 6–12 weeks.
- It is standard practice to give the vaccine into the left upper arm so that BCG status can be easily checked. The injection leaves a characteristic scar for life.
- Traumatic catheterization during bladder instillation of BCG may lead to systemic BCG infection. This usually responds well to antituberculous drugs.

DIPHTHERIA VACCINE

Class: Toxoid vaccine

Indications
* Prophylaxis of diphtheria.

Mechanism of action
* Diphtheria vaccine contains inactivated diphtheria toxin (toxoid), which stimulates production of antibodies. These provide immunity against *Corynebacterium diphtheriae*. The toxin is combined with aluminium to improve antigenicity.
* The diphtheria vaccine is only available as a combination product with other vaccines.

Adverse effects
* *Common*: pain and swelling at the site of injection.
* *Rare*: fever, arthralgia.

Contraindications
* Acute febrile illness.
* Severe reaction to a previous dose.

Interactions
* None.

Route of administration
* IM, deep SC.

Note
* The vaccine is given to children as part of a combination containing tetanus, pertussis and inactivated poliomyelitis. Some preparations contain Hib in addition. Treatment of Diphtheria is with anti-toxin and antibiotics i.e. erythromycin, penicillin.
* Diphtheria vaccine is also given to travellers going to areas where diphtheria is prevalent; the vaccine includes tetanus and inactivated poliomyelitis.
* Adults and children over 10 years of age who require a primary dose or a booster should be given the low-dose diphtheria vaccine combination, which includes tetanus and inactivated poliomyelitis. Diphtheria is an infection of the respiratory tract associated with formation of a membrane that may cause compromise of the airway. Symptoms are usually associated with lymphadenopathy and cutaneous diphtheria. Complications include neurological (neuropathies and muscle weakness) and cardiac (dysrhythmias, myocarditis, cardiomyopathy) involvement.

HAEMOPHILUS INFLUENZAE TYPE B (HIB) VACCINE

Class: Inactivated vaccine

Indications
* Prophylaxis of Hib infections.

Mechanism of action
* Hib vaccine contains a capsular polysaccharide obtained from Hib, which has been conjugated to a protein carrier (this enhances immunogenicity). Administration stimulates an antibody response.

Adverse effects
* *Common*: local erythema, fever.
* *Rare*: diarrhoea, vomiting, anaphylaxis.

Contraindications
* Acute febrile illness.
* Severe reaction to a previous dose.
* Pregnancy.
* Breastfeeding.

Interactions
* None.

Route of administration
* IM, deep SC.

Note
* The goal of vaccination is to prevent Hib epiglottitis, meningitis and pneumonia.
* Hib vaccine is not usually required for children over 4 years of age because the risk of infection with Hib falls rapidly after this age. Exceptions to this rule are patients with sickle-cell disease, asplenic patients and those receiving chemotherapy for malignancy.

HEPATITIS B VACCINE

Class: Subunit vaccine

Indications
* Prophylaxis of hepatitis B.

Mechanism of action
* The vaccine contains hepatitis B surface antigen (HBsAg), which is prepared in yeast by recombinant DNA technology. It stimulates production of anti-HBsAg antibodies, which confer protective immunity.

Adverse effects
* *Common*: discomfort at the injection site.
* *Rare*: anaphylaxis, thrombocytopenia.

Contraindications
* Acute febrile illness.
* Severe reaction to a previous dose.

Interactions
* None.

Route of administration
* IM (deltoid muscle, not gluteal as vaccine efficacy reduced), SC (to avoid bleeding in haemophilia patients).

Note
* Hepatitis B vaccine should be given to those at high risk (e.g. healthcare workers, haemophiliacs, babies born to infected mothers).
* The vaccine course involves 3 injections given at 0, 1 and 6 months. An accelerated course of 0, 1 and 2 months or 0, 7 and 21 days is possible but a booster at 1 year is recommended after an accelated course.
* Following a single episode of exposure to hepatitis B virus (e.g. contact with infected blood), in unimmunized individuals an injection of hepatitis B-specific immunoglobulin with the hepatitis B vaccine should be given as soon as possible. This confers a significant level of protection against the disease. A vaccine course may give lifelong immunity but a further booster at 5 years is recommended for health professionals. Individuals who fail to respond i.e. antibody titre less than 100 mIU/ml should have a booster, in some cases a repeat course is required.

HUMAN PAPILLOMA VIRUS (HPV) VACCINE

Class: Inactivated vaccine

Indications
- Prevention of cervical cancer.

Mechanism of action
- HPV types 16 and 18 are involved in the development of cervical cancer and vaccination reduces the risk significantly.

Adverse effects
- *Common*: injection site reactions.
- *Rare*: fever, diarrhoea, dizziness, myalgia, arthralgia.

Contraindications
- Acute febrile illness.

Interactions
- None.

Route of administration
- IM.

Note
- The vaccine is most effective if given before sexual activity starts.
- First dose given to girls aged 12–13 years, the second and third doses 1–2 months and 6 months after the first dose.
- Despite vaccination, cervical screening must continue as there are strains of HPV not covered by the vaccines.
- Currently only one of the two brands available prevents against cervical cancer and genital warts.

INFLUENZA VACCINE

Class: Inactivated vaccine

Indications
* Prevention of influenza and its complications.

Mechanism of action
* The influenza virus is constantly changing its external components called haemagglutinins and neuraminidases. It is important the vaccine in use contains the same H and N components to the prevalent strain. This is regulated by the World Health Organization, who advise which strains should be used in the vaccine.
* It takes 10–14 days to produce an antibody response to the vaccine.

Adverse effects
* *Common*: swelling at injection site.
* *Rare*: neurological disorders.

Contraindications
* Egg allergy.
* Acute febrile illness.

Interactions
* None.

Route of administration
* IM.

Note
* Immunization is recommended for:
    * Those aged 65 years or over.
    * Those aged over 6 months with chronic lung, heart, liver, kidney or neurological disease.
    * Those with Diabetes mellitus.
    * Those immunosuppressed because of treatment or disease.
* Healthcare workers should be vaccinated as an adjunct to good infection control procedures.

MENINGOCOCCAL GROUP C VACCINE

Class: Conjugate or polysaccharide vaccine

Indications
* Prophylaxis of *Neisseria meningitidis* serogroup C meningitis.

Mechanism of action
* The vaccine contains group C-specific meningococcal polysaccharides, which stimulate the immune system to produce protective antibodies.

Adverse effects
* *Common*: erythema and swelling at the site of injection, fever, headache.
* *Rare*: seizures, hypersensitivity, meningism.

Contraindications
* Acute febrile illness.
* Severe reaction to a previous dose.

Interactions
* None.

Route of administration
* IM, SC.

Note
* 40% of cases of meningitis are caused by group C *Neisseria meningitidis*, the remaining 60% being caused by group B strain.
* There are two types of meningococcal C vaccine in use:
  1. Group C conjugate vaccine: a conjugate between a protein carrier and group C-specific capsular polysaccharide.
  2. Polysaccharide vaccine: a combination of group C-specific polysaccharides.
* Meningococcal vaccine should be given to patients up to the age of 24 years who have not been previously immunized. As the risk of meningitis declines with age, immunization is not usually indicated in those over 25 years.
* Meningococcal vaccine should also be given to those with an absent or dysfunctional spleen (conjugate vaccine).
* Travellers to high-risk countries (e.g. Africa, Saudi Arabia) should be offered the meningococcal polysaccharide vaccine.

MEASLES, MUMPS, RUBELLA (MMR) VACCINE

Class: Combined live-attenuated vaccine

Indications
* Prophylaxis of measles, mumps and rubella.

Mechanism of action
* MMR vaccine contains live-attenuated strains of MMR viruses.
* It provides active immunity by stimulating an antibody-mediated response.

Adverse effects
* *Common*: fever, malaise, rash.
* *Rare*: parotid swelling, idiopathic thrombocytopenic purpura.

Contraindications
* Immunocompromised children.
* Pregnancy.
* Another live vaccine within the previous 3 weeks.
* Allergy to neomycin or kanamycin (MMR vaccine contains traces of both).
* Acute febrile illness.
* Severe reaction to a previous dose.
* Chemo/radiotherapy (defer the vaccine for 6 weeks).
* Leukaemia.
* Malignant conditions of the reticuloendothelial system.

Interactions
* None.

Route of administration
* IM, deep SC.

Note
* Women should avoid pregnancy for 1 month following MMR vaccination.
* Every child should receive 2 doses of the MMR unless there is a contraindication.
* Adverse effects commonly occur following the 1st dose and much less so following the 2nd dose of MMR vaccine.
* The link between MMR vaccine and both autism and inflammatory bowel disease has been disproved.
* MMR vaccine should be administered irrespective of previous infection with MMR.

PERTUSSIS VACCINE

Class: Inactivated vaccine

Indications
- Prophylaxis of whooping cough.

Mechanism of action
- Pertussis vaccine contains killed *Bordetella pertussis* organisms.
The vaccine induces active immunity by formation of antibodies
against *Bordetella pertussis*.

Adverse effects
- *Common*: fever, pain and redness at the site of injection.
- *Rare*: encephalopathy, convulsions, oedema and induration of the
limb into which the injection was given.

Contraindications
- Acute febrile illness.
- Severe reaction to a previous dose.

Interactions
- None.

Route of administration
- IM, deep SC.

Note
- Pertussis vaccine is given as a combination with other vaccines
(diptheria, tetanus, polio and haemophilus influenzae type B) at 2, 3,
4 months of age and then a school booster aged 3-5 years to reduce
the number of shots given to children. Some individuals can develop
whooping cough despite vaccination as the effects wane over the
years, however whooping cough is not deemed a serious condition
in older children and adults.
- Macrolide antibiotics e.g. erythromycin given early in the course
of whooping cough can reduce the severity of symptoms and
shorten the infectious period.

POLIOMYELITIS VACCINE

Class: Live-attenuated or inactivated vaccine

Indications

* Prophylaxis of poliomyelitis.

Mechanism of action

* The oral poliomyelitis vaccine (Sabin vaccine) contains live-attenuated strains of polioviruses. It induces active immunity by formation of IgG and IgA antibodies, thereby conferring protection against poliomyelitis infections of the CNS and GI tract.
* The inactivated subcutaneous vaccine (Salk vaccine) induces the formation of IgG antibodies and to a lesser extent IgA antibodies. It induces only a little immunity in the intestinal tract but confers protection against polio infections of the CNS.

Adverse effects

* *Rare*: paralysis with oral vaccine (less than 1 in 2 million doses).

Contraindications

* Sabin vaccine (oral):
    * Vomiting and diarrhoea.
    * Immunosuppression.
    * Pregnancy.
    * Severe reaction to a previous dose.
    * Malignancy.
    * Receiving chemotherapy and/or radiotherapy (defer the vaccine for 6 months).

Interactions

* None.

Route of administration

* Salk vaccine: SC.
* Sabin vaccine: oral.

Note

* The inactivated vaccine is recommended for routine immunization.
* The inactivated poliomyelitis vaccine comes as a combination product with other vaccines, which is used for the primary immunization and boosters.
* Poliomyelitis is endemic in developing countries and therefore non-immunized travellers should be vaccinated with the inactivated vaccine with 3 doses. Those who have not been vaccinated in the last 10 years should have a booster dose of the combination vaccine including diphtheria, tetanus and inactivated poliomyelitis.
* After the primary course of vaccines booster doses are only recommended for adults at risk, e.g. travellers and healthcare workers every 10 years.
* Orally vaccinated children are usually infectious to others for about 6 weeks due to shedding of the virus in the faeces.

TETANUS VACCINE

Class: Toxoid vaccine

Indications
- Prophylaxis of tetanus.

Mechanism of action
- Tetanus vaccine contains inactivated tetanus toxin (toxoid), which stimulates antibody-mediated active immunity.

Adverse effects
- *Common*: pain and tenderness at the site of injection.
- *Rare*: fever.

Contraindications
- Acute febrile illness.
- Severe reaction to a previous dose.

Interactions
- None.

Route of administration
- IM.

Note
- Tetanus vaccine comes as a combination product with other vaccines, including diphtheria, pertussis and inactivated poliomyelitis.
- A full course of tetanus immunization should be given to both non-immunized individuals and to those with unknown immunization status following a penetrating injury or burns (three combination vaccines given monthly and a booster every 10 years).
- Following an injury in a previously immunized individual, a booster should be given only if more than 10 years have elapsed since the last administration. Tetanus is treated with human tetanus immunoglobulin, diazepam is given for the muscle spasms but in serious cases in order to control the spasms patients are paralysed and put on a ventilator.

OBSTETRICS AND GYNAECOLOGY

Management guidelines

CONTRACEPTION
* A total of 90% of fertile young females who have regular unprotected intercourse become pregnant within 1 year.

Methods of contraception
* *Natural methods*: rhythm method, coitus interruptus.
* *Barrier methods*: male or female condom, diaphragm, cervical cap.
* *IUCD*: this method is unsuitable for women with heavy or painful periods. IUCDs usually last a minimum of 5 years.
* *Mirena device*: a progesterone-loaded IUCD, especially useful for women with heavy periods.
* *Hormonal*: COC pill, progestogen-only pill (POP), subcutaneous medroxyprogesterone depot injection (usually lasts 8–12 weeks), subcutaneous implant (usually lasts 3–5 years).
* *Sterilization*: vasectomy in males (failure rate of about 1 in 2000), laparoscopic occlusion of the fallopian tubes in females (failure rate of about 1 in 200).

Risks and benefits of the combined oral contraceptive pill (COC) pill
* Giving oestrogens alone involves a risk of developing breast cancer or endometrial cancer in women with a uterus. For this reason, oestrogen is combined with a progestogen in the COC pill.

The Hands–on Guide to Clinical Pharmacology, 3rd Edition. By S Chatu.
Published 2010 by Blackwell Publishing Ltd.

- Oestrogen can also predispose to thromboembolic events. Women who are obese, diabetic, smoke or have any other additional risk factors for thromboembolic events should either be warned about the risks or should be declined the COC pill, if appropriate.
- The COC pill furthermore protects against pelvic infection/ pelvic inflammatory disease (PID), ovarian cancer, ovarian cysts and benign breast disease.

Progestogen-only pill (POP), ('mini-pill')
- The POP is given when COCs are contraindicated (e.g. history of thromboembolic disease). However, the POP has a slightly higher failure rate than the COC pill.
- The POP must be taken at the same time each day. The contraceptive effect is inadequate if administration is delayed by more than 3 hours. In this case the pill should be continued as normal, but a different method of contraception (e.g. condom) should be used for a period of 1 week.

Post-coital contraception
- 'Morning-after pill' (contains levonorgestrel) – give one dose within 72 hours following unprotected sexual intercourse, followed by a second dose 12 hours later.
- Alternatively, an IUCD can be placed within 5 days following unprotected intercourse.

HORMONE REPLACEMENT THERAPY (HRT)
- *Climacteric*: this is the time of waning fertility leading up to the menopause.
- *Menopause*: the time of the last menstrual cycle; average age in the UK is 51 years.
- *Premature menopause*: this occurs in about 1% of women in the UK, and is defined as the last menstrual cycle occurring before the age of 40 years.
- HRT consists of regular oestrogen and progesterone given for a period of up to 5 years once the menopause has been reached. It can be given orally or as a patch, gel or SC implant. HRT aims to counter the changes brought on by the menopause, which are due to a lack of oestrogens. It should not be given for any other reason than to relieve post-menopausal symptoms.
- Women on HRT need to be reviewed yearly to assess the need for ongoing HRT.

Benefits of HRT
- Symptomatic relief of post-menopausal symptoms (e.g. flushing, sweating, mood changes, thinning hair, wrinkling skin).
- Prevention of menopause-associated disease processes (e.g. osteoporosis, ovarian cancer).
- A progestogen is added to HRT in order to prevent cystic hyperplasia and oestrogen-related cancer of the endometrium.

Disadvantages of HRT
- Adverse effects of oestrogen and progestogen.
- Increased risk of breast cancer.
- Recent evidence suggests an increased risk of IHD and dementia.

Contraindications to HRT
- Pregnancy and breastfeeding.
- Oestrogen-dependent cancer (such as endometrial and breast cancer).
- Thromboembolic disorders.
- Liver disease.
- Undiagnosed vaginal bleeding.

HYPERTENSION IN PREGNANCY
- Admit if BP exceeds 160/100 mmHg in a known hypertensive.
- Advise bed rest.
- Monitor BP 2–4-hourly, urine protein by urinalysis, plasma urate and LFTs, platelet count and the fetus cardiotocography CTG.
- If high BP persists, treat with antihypertensives (see below).
- If high BP persists with proteinuria, treat as for pre-eclampsia.

Pharmacological treatment
- Treat if BP reaches 160/100 mmHg.
- Drugs that are commonly used:
  1. Oral methyldopa.
  2. Oral beta blocker (e.g. labetalol).
  3. Oral nifedipine.

INDUCTION OF LABOUR
- Assess the state of the cervix prior to induction using the Bishop score (this assesses station, position and cervical effacement/consistency/dilatation).
- Unripe cervix must be ripened with vaginal prostaglandins (e.g. PGE_2).
- If this fails, consider Caesarean section.
- Once the cervix is ripe, rupture the membranes.
- Monitor fetal heart with CTG.
- If necessary, give IV oxytocin until effective uterine contractions are present (sometimes given until delivery).
- A combination of IM ergometrine and oxytocin is given to the mother when the baby's anterior shoulder is delivered. This accelerates the third stage of labour and reduces the risk of post-partum haemorrhage.
- NB: an induction should always be managed as high-risk labour.

MENORRHAGIA
- Treat any underlying cause (e.g. pelvic pathology, clotting disorder, medical disorders).
- In most cases no organic cause is found (termed dysfunctional uterine bleeding) and treatment is mainly symptomatic:

- Medical treatment:
  - To decrease blood loss: antifibrinolytics (e.g. tranexamic acid), NSAIDs (e.g. mefenamic acid) or systemic progestogens.
  - To restore a regular cycle: COC pill.
- Progesterone-loaded IUCD (Mirena):
- Surgical treatment:
  - Endometrial resection or ablation.
  - Myomectomy for fibroids (only performed if further pregnancies are desired or patient is unwilling to have hysterectomy, as the complication rate of myomectomy is greater than that of hysterectomy).
  - Hysterectomy in severe cases.

POLYCYSTIC OVARY SYNDROME

- Prevalence is about 20–30% of women, but only 10% are symptomatic and therefore may need treatment.
- Encourage weight loss, if appropriate.
- For regulation of menstruation: COC pill.
- For hirsutism/acne:
  - COC pill containing cyproterone acetate.
  - Alternatively, hirsutism may be treated by depilation (waxing), electrolysis or laser hair removal.
- If pregnancy is desired:
  - Clomiphene (an oestrogen antagonist acting on the hypothalamus) – this induces ovulation in about 70% of women given clomiphene.
  - If clomiphene fails, consider gonadotrophins.
- NB: it is important to monitor serum or urine oestrogen levels to detect any developing ovarian hyperstimulation.

PRE-ECLAMPSIA

- The objective of treatment is to prevent eclampsia.
- Admit if BP is > 140/90 mmHg with proteinuria and oedema.
- Monitor BP 2–4-hourly, 24-hour urine protein, plasma urate, platelets and LFTs (especially ALT, AST), and the fetus (CTG).
- If BP is > 150/100 mmHg, control with antihypertensives to prevent maternal intracranial haemorrhage: IV hydralazine or IV labetalol or oral nifedipine.
- Advise bed rest.
- The mother must be monitored after delivery, as eclampsia can occur post partum (especially within the first 48 hours).
- Beware of warning signs of eclampsia: epigastric pain, headaches, blurred vision.

ECLAMPSIA (MATERNAL CONVULSIONS DURING PREGNANCY)

- Lie the patient on her left side.
- Give oxygen.

- Give IV magnesium sulphate to control fits.
- Give IV hydralazine or IV labetalol to control BP.
- Once BP and fits are controlled, deliver the baby.
- Check magnesium levels, test patellar reflexes regularly and monitor urine output after giving magnesium sulphate (loss of reflexes is an early sign of toxicity; magnesium sulphate is excreted in the urine).
- The mother must be monitored after delivery, as eclampsia can occur post partum (especially within the first 48 hours).
- *Note*: delivery is the only cure.

Drugs

ERGOMETRINE

Class: Ergot alkaloid

Indications
*   Prevention and treatment of post-partum haemorrhage.
*   Active management of the third stage of labour.
*   Uterine bleeding due to an incomplete abortion.

Mechanism of action
*   Exact mechanism is not fully understood.
*   It may act at alpha adrenoceptors, prostaglandin and serotonin receptors in smooth muscle.
*   Ergometrine causes uterine contractions and has some degree of vasoconstrictor action.

Adverse effects
*   *Common*: nausea, vomiting, abdominal pain, hypertension, headache, dizziness.
*   *Rare*: palpitations, tingling in fingers, anginal pain.

Contraindications
*   Induction of labour.
*   First and second stages of labour.
*   Eclampsia.
*   Hypertension.
*   PVD and IHD (due to vasoconstrictor action).
*   Severe cardiac, hepatic or renal impairment.
*   Sepsis.

Interactions
*   *Macrolide antibiotics*: increased risk of ergotism (nausea, vomiting, visual disturbances, peripheral ischaemia).
*   *Protease inhibitors*: increased risk of ergotism.
*   *Tetracycline*: increased risk of ergotism.

Route of administration
*   Oral, IM, IV (in emergencies).

Note
*   IM ergometrine is often given together with oxytocin in the third stage of labour or in post-partum haemorrhage. These two drugs, when combined, are more effective than either one of them alone.
*   Owing to its vasoconstrictor action, ergometrine may cause spasm of the coronary arteries, resulting in anginal pain.
*   Ergometrine will cause an inappropriately relaxed uterus to contract, aiming to reduce bleeding from the placental bed. It exerts little effect on an already contracted uterus.

OESTROGENS

Class: Sex hormones

Indications

* Contraception (in the form of the COC pill).
* HRT.
* Atrophic vaginitis (topical use only).

Mechanism of action

* In HRT, replacing the deficient oestrogen alleviates menopausal symptoms.
* Given as the COC pill, oestrogens inhibit the release of follicle-stimulating hormone (FSH) from the anterior pituitary by negative feedback. This prevents maturation of the Graafian follicle in the ovary.

Adverse effects

* *Common*: fluid retention, hypertension, loss of libido, nausea, vomiting, breast tenderness, weight gain, acne, mood swings, worsening of pre-existing migraine.
* *Rare*: thromboembolic events, headache, depression, slightly increased risk of breast cancer, slightly increased risk of endometrial cancer (only if given alone without a progestogen), hepatic tumours, cholestatic jaundice.

Contraindications

* Pregnancy.
* Breastfeeding.
* Previous thromboembolic events (e.g. PE).
* Active hepatic disease (oestrogens are metabolized by the liver).
* Oestrogen-dependent tumours (e.g. endometrial cancer).
* Focal migraine.

Interactions

* *Broad-spectrum antibiotics*: these may decrease the effects of oestrogens by impairing the gut flora responsible for recycling ethinyloestradiol in the large bowel
* *Carbamazepine*: this increases the metabolism of oestrogens, thereby decreasing their effect.
* *Phenytoin, rifampicin*: these drugs decrease the plasma concentration of oestrogens.
* *Warfarin*: oestrogens reduce the anticoagulant effect of warfarin.

Route of administration

* HRT: oral, transdermal patch, SC implant, gel.
* Contraception: oral, SC, IM.
* Atrophic vaginitis: vaginal cream or pessary.

Note

* BP should be checked regularly due to the risk of hypertension.
* The COC pill failure rate is 3–5 pregnancies per 100 woman-years of administration. This is largely due to incorrect self-administration.
* Oestrogens may need to be discontinued several weeks prior to surgery, as they predispose to thromboembolic events. Vomiting and diarrhoea can interfere with pill absorption hence additional precautions e.g. condoms should be used during and for 7 days after.

OXYTOCIN

Class: Oxytocic agent

Indications
* Induction or augmentation of labour.
* Management of the third stage of labour.
* Prevention and treatment of post-partum haemorrhage.
* Uterine bleeding after spontaneous or induced abortion.

Mechanism of action
* Oxytocin produces contractions of the fundus in the pregnant uterus by acting on local oxytocin receptors.
* It also enhances uterine contractions by increasing the production of prostaglandins in the myometrium.

Adverse effects
* *Common*: uterine spasm, nausea, vomiting.
* *Rare*: fluid and electrolyte disturbance, hypotension, tachycardia, cardiac dysrhythmias.

Contraindications
* Mechanical obstruction in labour and any other condition where vaginal delivery is not advisable.
* Predisposition to uterine rupture (e.g. previous Caesarean section).
* Fetal distress.

Interactions
* *Sympathomimetics*: concomitant use increases risk of hypertension due to the enhanced vasopressor effect.

Route of administration
* IV.

Note
* Careful monitoring of fetal heart rate and uterine contractions is required when oxytocin is used in labour. This is due to the risk of fetal hypoxia caused by uterine hyperstimulation. Oxytocin should be discontinued in cases of uterine hyperactivity or fetal distress.
* Oxytocin is often given together with ergometrine in the third stage of labour or in post-partum haemorrhage. These two drugs, when combined, are more effective than either one of them alone.
* Oxytocin is infused using IV fluids. If large amounts of oxytocin, and therefore fluids, are given, the patient may suffer hyponatraemic seizures secondary to water intoxication. This risk is increased by oxytocin's antidiuretic activity (it structurally resembles vasopressin).

PROGESTOGENS

Class: Sex hormones

Indications
* Contraception.
* Part of HRT.
* Menstrual disorders (e.g. dysmenorrhoea, menorrhagia).
* Endometriosis.
* Neoplastic disease (endometrial cancer, renal cell carcinoma, second- or third-line therapy in the treatment of breast cancer).

Mechanism of action
* The main contraceptive effect of progestogens is due to their action on cervical mucus, which is rendered impenetrable to sperm. Progestogens also prevent implantation of the fertilized ovum by rendering the endometrium hostile.
* Progestogens immobilize sperm by increasing the pH of uterine fluid.
* Progestogens also suppress the secretion of gonadotrophins from the anterior pituitary by negative feedback, thus inhibiting ovulation in about 40% of females.
* In endometriosis, progestogens are used to inhibit menstruation, thus producing regression of small lesions.

Adverse effects
* *Common*: menstrual irregularities, breast tenderness, weight gain, acne, bloating, nausea, vomiting, hot flushes.
* *Rare*: cholestatic jaundice, thromboembolism.

Contraindications
* Pregnancy.
* Severe hypertension.
* Unexplained vaginal bleeding.
* Hepatic impairment.

Interactions
* *Rifamycins*: reduced contraceptive effect.
* *Carbamazepine, phenytoin*: these drugs reduce the contraceptive effect.
* *Ciclosporin*: progestogens increase the plasma concentration of ciclosporin.
* *Warfarin*: reduced anticoagulant effect.

Route of administration
* Oral, vaginal gel/pessary, rectal, IM, SC implant, IUCD.

Note
* Progestogens are divided into two main classes:
  * Progesterone with its analogues (hydroxyprogesterone, dydrogesterone, medroxyprogesterone)
  * Testosterone with its analogues (norgestrel, norethisterone). Gestodene, desogestrel and norgestimate are derivatives of norgestrel.

TRANEXAMIC ACID

Class: Antifibrinolytic agent

Indications
- Menorrhagia.
- Treatment and prevention of haemorrhage (e.g. haemophilia, perioperatively).
- Hereditary angioedema. Treatment of epistaxis

Mechanism of action
- Tranexamic acid inhibits activation of plasminogen to plasmin, which is an essential factor in the fibrinolysis cascade. This action enhances clot stability.
- Tranexamic acid has no effect on platelets.

Adverse effects
- *Rare*: hypotension, thromboembolic events (including central retinal artery and vein obstruction), colour vision disturbance, dizziness.
- *Common*: nausea, vomiting, diarrhoea

Contraindications
- Thromboembolic disease e.g. DVT, PE.

Interactions
- None known.

Route of administration
- Oral, IV.

Note
- Tranexamic acid is used in dental, gynaecological and urological surgery in patients who have clotting disorders (e.g. von Willebrand's disease, haemophilia). It is not used in abdominal or thoracic surgery due to the risk of insoluble haematomas forming. For menorrhagia treatment is commenced on intitation for up to 4 days.
- Patients should be made aware of the symptoms of arterial or venous thromboembolism which can rarely occur with tranexamic acid.

Related drugs
- Aminocaproic acid, aprotinin.

ANAESTHESIA

General anaesthesia (pp. 207–208)
Premedication
Anaesthetic agents
Muscle-relaxing agents
Analgesic agents

Regional (local) anaesthesia (p. 208–209)
Local infiltration
Bier's block
Epidural anaesthesia
Spinal anaesthesia

Drugs (pp. 210–216)
Anticholinesterases (edrophonium, neostigmine,)
Inhalational agents (desflurane, enflurane, isoflurane, sevoflurane)
Lidocaine
Nitrous oxide
Non-depolarizing muscle relaxants (atracurium, mivacurium,
pancuronium, rocuronium, vecuronium)
Propofol
Suxamethonium

General anaesthesia

- General anaesthetic agents are employed as an adjunct to surgical procedures. They achieve a state of complete but reversible loss of consciousness in which the patient is unaware of and unresponsive to painful stimuli.

    Unlike local anaesthetics, general anaesthetics are given systemically. They produce their effects by acting on the CNS, while maintaining the function of other body systems such as the cardiovascular and respiratory systems.
- Agents used in general anaesthesia are legion and can be divided into the following four categories.

Premedication (given before induction of general anaesthesia)
- Benzodiazepines to reduce anxiety.
- Antimuscarinics (e.g. hyoscine, atropine), which inhibit the parasympathetic nervous system to reduce bronchial secretions,

The Hands–on Guide to Clinical Pharmacology, 3rd Edition. By S Chatu.
Published 2010 by Blackwell Publishing Ltd.

salivation and vagal reflexes (bradycardia, myocardial depression) to facilitate general anaesthesia.
* Opioids for analgesic and sedative effects (give with an antiemetic).
* Note: the use of premedication is declining.

Anaesthetic agents
* Induction of general anaesthesia by IV agents:
    * Non-barbiturates (propofol, ketamine, etomidate).
    * Barbiturates (thiopentone).
* Maintenance of anaesthesia by inhalational agents (e.g. isoflurane, sevoflurane, desflurane), but sometimes achieved with IV propofol alone (total IV anaesthesia).
* Can use certain inhalational agents for induction and maintenance (sevoflurane is commonly used in children).

Muscle-relaxing agents
* Suxamethonium is a depolarizing muscle relaxant mainly used to aid tracheal intubation because of its rapid onset of action and short duration.
* Non-depolarizing (e.g. atracurium) muscle relaxants are used to facilitate certain surgical procedures (e.g. laparotomy, neurosurgery) and prevent any resistance on a ventilator.
* After surgery, the effects of non-depolarizing muscle relaxants are reversed by anticholinesterase drugs (edrophonium, neostigmine).

Analgesic agents (used perioperatively)
* Paracetamol.
* NSAIDs, e.g. diclofenac, ibuprofen.
* Opioids in conjunction with an antiemetic.
* Local anaesthetics (lidocaine, bupivacaine).

Regional (local) anaesthesia

* Local anaesthesia is the method of choice for many minor surgical procedures. It is especially useful in patients suffering from severe cardiorespiratory disease who are more susceptible to the risks of general anaesthesia.
* Agents used to induce local anaesthesia (e.g. lidocaine) act by causing a local nerve conduction block. The following types of local anaesthesia are used:
    1. Local infiltration.
    2. Nerve block (e.g. ring block in a finger).
    3. Local IV regional anaesthesia (Bier's block).
    4. Central neural blockade (epidural/spinal anaesthesia).

Bier's block
* This technique provides good operating conditions for hand surgery or manual reduction of wrist/forearm fractures.
* A tourniquet is applied to the upper arm and inflated to 300 mmHg.

- Local anaesthetic (prilocaine) is then injected IV into the arm, distal to the tourniquet. This produces whole arm analgesia rather than blockade of individual nerves.
- Tourniquet is deflated after 20 minutes.

Epidural anaesthesia

- Used in obstetrics for pain relief in labour and during Caesarean section and other surgical intervention. Can be used for post-operative analgesia when the epidural catheter is left in.
- In this technique, local anaesthetic (bupivacaine with or without diamorphine) is injected into the extradural space of the spinal cord via a thin catheter. It then diffuses through the nerve sheaths into the cerebrospinal fluid (CSF).
- A great advantage of epidural anaesthesia is that the catheter can be left *in situ*, thus enabling continuous infusion of local anaesthetic.
- Epidural anaesthesia blocks spinal roots but inadvertently causes sympathetic nerve blockade in the region of infiltration that supplies the blood vessels, leading to vasodilatation and hence hypotension. This can be corrected with IV fluids and/or a vasoconstrictor such as ephedrine. Other vasoconstrictors can also be used (metaraminol, phenylephrine).

Spinal anaesthesia

- Used in the elderly who are deemed high risk for a general anaesthetic because of cardiorespiratory, renal or liver problems, for surgery below the umbilicus.
- In this technique, local anaesthetic (bupivacaine) is injected directly into the CSF around the spinal cord at the lumbar region where the spinal cord ends into the subarachnoid space. The onset of action is therefore faster than with epidural anaesthesia and a smaller dose is needed to achieve the desired effect.
- Spinal anaesthesia wears off after 3–4 hours.
- Spinal anaesthesia blocks spinal roots but inadvertently causes sympathetic nerve blockade in the region of infiltration that supplies the blood vessels, leading to vasodilatation and hence hypotension. This can be corrected with IV fluids and/or a vasoconstrictor such as ephedrine. Other vasoconstrictors can also be used (metaraminol, phenylephrine).

Drugs

ANTICHOLINESTERASES

(Edrophonium, neostigmine)

Class: Anticholinesterase

Indications
* Reversal of non-depolarizing muscle relaxants.

Mechanism of action
* These drugs inhibit the enzyme acetylcholinesterase in the synaptic cleft of neuromuscular junctions. This leads to a build-up of acetylcholine in the synaptic cleft, thereby reversing the effects of the non-depolarizing muscle relaxants that are competitive agonists. This enhances neurotransmission, leading to loss of paralysis.

Adverse effects
* *Common*: abdominal cramps, hypersalivation, diarrhoea, bradycardia (all due to excessive muscarinic effects as a result of acetylcholine stimulating muscarinic receptors in the heart, smooth muscle and glands).

Contraindications
* Intestinal obstruction.
* Urinary obstruction.

Interactions
* *Aminoglycosides*: antagonize the effects of neostigmine.
* *Clindamycin*: antagonizes the effects of neostigmine.
* *Lithium*: antagonizes the effects of neostigmine.

Route of administration
* IV (for reversal of non-depolarizing muscle relaxants).

Note
* Neostigmine has a short duration of action (2–4 hours).
* Adverse effects of neostigmine, such as bradycardia and excessive salivation, can be counteracted by an antimuscarinic agent (e.g. atropine or glycopyrronium).
* Neostigmine is used more often than edrophonium to reverse muscle relaxants.
* Neuromuscular transmission may be impaired if excessive doses of neostigmine are given due to a depolarizing block. This leads to a cholinergic crisis when excess acetylcholine impairs muscle function causing muscle fasciculations, sweating and excessive salivation. Treatment requires an anticholinergic such as atropine.

Related drugs
* Distigmine, pyridostigmine (only used in the treatment of myasthenia gravis).
* Edrophonium (used in tensilon test and occasionally used to reverse non-depolarizing muscle relaxants).

INHALATIONAL GENERAL ANAESTHETIC AGENTS

(Desflurane, enflurane, isoflurane, sevoflurane)

Class: Inhalational general anaesthetic

Indications
- Maintenance of anaesthesia.
- Induction and maintenance in children – sevoflurane.

Mechanism of action
- Exact mechanism is not fully understood.
- Most theories infer that general anaesthetic agents act on the cell membrane in the CNS.
- Three important theories have been put forward:

   1. *Lipid theory*: anaesthetics change the lipid component of cell membranes and thus alter transmembrane ion movements to produce anaesthesia.

   2. *Protein theory*: anaesthetics bind to proteins and reversibly change their structure to induce anaesthesia.

   3. *Hydrate theory*: anaesthetics produce crystals within cell membranes by freezing the water component of the membrane, thus producing anaesthesia.

Adverse effects
- *Common*: respiratory depression, hypotension, tachycardia.
- *Rare*: hepatotoxicity.

Contraindications
- Hypersensitivity.
- Malignant hyperpyrexia.

Interactions
- *Antihypertensives*: enhance the hypotensive effect of general anaesthetics.
- *Epinephrine*: risk of possible cardiac dysrhythmias if given with a general anaesthetic.
- *MAOIs, TCAs*: increased risk of arrhythmias and hypotension with a general anaesthetic.

Route of administration
- Inhalation (via anaesthetic machine).

Note
- Volatile liquid anaesthetics require a carrier gas for administration. Nitrous oxide/oxygen mixtures, air and oxygen are all used for this purpose.
- Isoflurane is used in preference to halothane and enflurane as it has a much lower incidence of hepatotoxicity and little effect on cardiac output and BP.
- Coughing and breath-holding on induction with isoflurane due to its pungent odour precludes it use as an induction agent.

LIDOCAINE (LIGNOCAINE)

Class: Local anaesthetic; class I antiarrhythmic agent

Indications
- Local anaesthesia.
- Ventricular dysrhythmias (especially following MI).

Mechanism of action
- Lidocaine blocks fast sodium channels in nerve axons. This leads to the following:

   1. Inhibition of generation of action potentials thus causing a reversible nerve conduction block.

   2. Suppression of premature ventricular beats and ventricular tachycardia by slowing the conduction velocity along the Purkinje fibres and ventricular muscle in the heart.

Adverse effects
- *Common*: nausea, vomiting, drowsiness, dizziness, perioral tingling (all are signs of toxicity).
- *Rare*: cardiovascular toxicity: bradycardia, hypotension, cardiac arrest; CNS toxicity: convulsions, confusion, coma.

Contraindications
- IV administration is contraindicated in the following:
   - All degrees of AV node block and SA node disorders.
   - Severe cardiac failure.
   - Acute porphyria.

Interactions
- *Antiarrhythmics*: concomitant use increases the risk of myocardial depression.

Route of administration
- IV (dysrhythmias only); subdural, epidural; intradermal or SC injection at desired site; topical application to mucous membranes and skin.

Note
- Extreme care must be taken to avoid accidental IV injection during administration of local anaesthesia.
- Duration of local anaesthesia is prolonged when lidocaine is administered with epinephrine (due to local vasoconstriction).
- Solutions containing lidocaine and epinephrine must not be used in ring block anaesthesia (e.g. fingers, toes, penis) as this may cause ischaemic necrosis. Instead, solutions containing only lidocaine should be used.
- Lidocaine should not be injected into inflamed or infected tissue as this may cause systemic effects (due to rapid absorption from these sites).

Related drugs
- Bupivacaine, levobupivacaine, prilocaine, ropivacaine (all are purely local anaesthetics).

NITROUS OXIDE

Class: Inhalational agent

Indications
- Maintenance of anaesthesia (in combination with inhalational anaesthetic agents).
- Analgesia without loss of consciousness (e.g. in labour).

Mechanism of action
- Exact mechanism is not fully understood.
- Nitrous oxide may act through inhibition of both N-methyl-D-aspartate (NMDA) glutamate receptors and non-NMDA glutamate receptors in the CNS.

Adverse effects
- *Rare*: bone marrow suppression, megaloblastic anaemia by interfering with the action Vitamin B12 (both following prolonged exposure).

Contraindications
- Pneumothorax (air pockets in closed spaces may expand).
- Bowel obstruction.

Interactions
- *Methotrexate*: nitrous oxide increases the antifolate effect of methotrexate.

Route of administration
- Inhalation.

Note
- For analgesia during labour, nitrous oxide is used as a mixture of 50% oxygen and 50% nitrous oxide. This can be employed as patient-controlled analgesia (PCA).
- Nitrous oxide is not effective enough to be used on its own in surgery. However, it is widely used as a carrier gas for general anaesthesia in combination with other agents (e.g. isoflurane).
- Low blood solubility of nitrous oxide leads to rapid induction and recovery. Nitrous oxide has little effect on the cardiovascular or respiratory systems.

NON-DEPOLARIZING MUSCLE RELAXANTS

(Atracurium, rocuronium, vecuronium)

Class: Non-depolarizing muscle relaxant

Indications
*   To achieve muscle relaxation in general anaesthesia to facilitate certain surgical procedures, e.g. laparotomy.
*   In mechanical ventilation when paralysis is required.

Mechanism of action
*   These agents competitively bind to nicotinic acetylcholine receptors at motor end-plates of skeletal muscle, antagonizing the neurotransmitting action of acetylcholine. This causes paralysis of skeletal muscle. One major effect is immediate loss of spontaneous respiration, hence respiratory support is required until the drug is reversed with an anticholinesterase or until its effects terminate.

Adverse effects
*   *Common*: rash, flushing, hypotension.
*   *Rare*: anaphylactoid reaction, bronchospasm.

Contraindications
*   Hypersensitivity.

Interactions
*   *Aminoglycosides, clindamycin, piperacillin*: enhance the effects of non-depolarizing muscle relaxants.
*   *Lithium, IV magnesium, propranolol, nifedipine, verapamil*: enhance the effects of non-depolarizing muscle relaxants.
*   *Carbamazepine, phenytoin*: antagonize the effects of non-depolarizing muscle relaxants.

Route of administration
*   IV.

Note
*   Non-depolarizing muscle relaxants of short/intermediate duration of action (atracurium and vecuronium) are more widely used than those of long duration of action.
*   Atracurium has an intermediate duration of action (30–45 minutes), and its onset of action is within 1–3 minutes. Duration of action is prolonged in hypothermia and myasthenia gravis.
*   Non-depolarizing muscle relaxants are not thought to cause malignant hyperpyrexia and have no analgesic or sedative properties.
*   Once a muscle relaxant is given, ventilation should be supported as there will be spontaneous paralysis of the respiratory muscles. Muscle relaxants are only used in the context of a general anaesthetic.
*   The action of non-depolarizing agents is reversible with an anticholinesterase agent (neostigmine, edrophonium).
*   Atracurium is unique as it undergoes inactivation in the plasma and thus can be used in patients with hepatic or renal impairment.

Related drugs
*   Cisatracurium, mivacurium, pancuronium.

PROPOFOL

Class: Intravenous anaesthetic agent

Indications

- Induction of anaesthesia.
- Total intravenous anaesthesia.
- Sedation during diagnostic and surgical procedures.
- Sedation in intensive care.

Mechanism of action

- Exact mechanism is not fully understood.
- There is evidence to suggest that propofol may act at $GABA_A$ receptors in the CNS.

Adverse effects

- *Common*: bradycardia, apnoea, hypotension, pain on injection.
- *Rare*: anaphylaxis, convulsions, pulmonary oedema.

Contraindications

- None.

Interactions

- *ACE inhibitors*: enhance the hypotensive effect of propofol.
- *Beta blockers*: enhance the hypotensive effect of propofol.
- *Calcium-channel blockers*: enhance the hypotensive effect of propofol.
- *Neuroleptics*: enhance the hypotensive effects of propofol.

Route of administration

- IV.

Note

- Propofol is widely used due to its rapid recovery rate without any nausea and 'hangover' effect.
- Slow administration is recommended in the elderly and hypertensive patients, as a marked decrease in BP can occur with rapid administration.
- Propofol induces sleep in one arm–brain circulation time (3–5 seconds).
- The pain caused by IV injection can be reduced by infiltrating lidocaine into the injection site prior to administration.

SUXAMETHONIUM

Class: Depolarizing muscle relaxant

Indications
* Used to aid endotracheal intubation by relaxing muscles.

Mechanism of action
* Suxamethonium imitates the action of acetylcholine at the neuromuscular junction on nicotinic receptors in skeletal muscles. This causes a depolarizing block and rapid muscle paralysis within 1 minute. Effects last about 5 minutes but intermittent boluses can be given.
* Suxamethonium is rapidly inactivated by plasma cholinesterase, hence its duration of action is for a few minutes. In some patients there is a deficiency or abnormality of this enzyme and the block can last for hours, especially if given with medication that enhances the effects of suxamethonium.

Adverse effects
* *Common*: muscle pain from fasciculations, bradycardia.
* *Rare*: hyperkalaemia, malignant hyperpyrexia, anaphylaxis.

Contraindications
* History of malignant hyperpyrexia.
* Hyperkalaemia.
* Recent burns, severe muscle trauma, paraplegia (increased risk of hyperkalaemia).

Interactions
* *Propofol*: increased risk of bradycardia and myocardial depression.
* *Aminoglycosides, clindamycin, piperacillin, vancomycin*: enhance the effects of suxamethonium.
* *Propranolol, verapamil*: enhance the effects of suxamethonium.
* *Lithium, IV magnesium, metoclopramide, neostigmine*: enhance the effects of suxamethonium.

Route of administration
* IV.

Note
* Suxamethonium causes a transient rise in potassium, intracranial and intraocular pressure that is of no clinical significance in normal individuals.
* Muscle pains postoperatively are due to fasciculations that occur before the onset of paralysis with suxamethonium.
* Antimuscarinic, e.g. atropine, can be given to prevent stimulation of the muscarinic receptors (parasympathetic system) by suxamethonium, which causes effects on the heart, smooth muscle and increases secretions from glands.
* Suxamethonium does not produce unconsciousness, hence is contraindicated in conscious patients.

POISONING AND OVERDOSE

Management guidelines

AIMS OF TREATMENT
- Decrease absorption of the substance (give activated charcoal within 1 hour of ingestion orally or via nasogastric tube, perform gastric lavage or whole bowel irrigation).
- Increase elimination of the substance (e.g. alkalinization of the urine or haemodialysis).
- Give specific antidote where appropriate.

GENERAL MANAGEMENT
- Resuscitate the patient (Airway, Breathing, Circulation) if appropriate.
- Make every attempt to obtain a history (what, when, how much and route of exposure).
- Physical examination may give clues to substance taken (e.g. respiratory depression –opiates, benzodiazepines).
- If the substance is known, follow specific management as shown below.
- If the substance is not known, blood and urine samples should be taken for toxicology screen and 4-hourly paracetamol and salicylate levels should be taken and treat complications as they arise.

The Hands–on Guide to Clinical Pharmacology, 3rd Edition. By S Chatu.
Published 2010 by Blackwell Publishing Ltd.

- If specialist advice is needed, call the appropriate national or regional poison centre.
- Provide supportive treatment.
- Treat any complications (e.g. dysrhythmias, hypoxia, hypotension, convulsions, hypothermia).
- Those who have taken an overdose with medication that has a delayed action or is a modified release preparation who appear well should be admitted for monitoring, e.g. iron, paracetamol.
- If overdose was intentional, the patient should undergo a psychiatric assessment once recovered.

MANAGEMENT OF SOME COMMON SPECIFIC OVERDOSES/POISONS

Aspirin
- Measure plasma salicylate levels to guide treatment 4 hours after ingestion.
- Give activated charcoal if within 1 hour of ingestion orally or by nasogastric tube, provided not too drowsy as may vomit and aspirate.
- Replace fluid and electrolyte losses.
- Elimination is increased by urinary alkalinization, achieved by administrating IV sodium bicarbonate.
- In severe overdose, i.e. levels more than 5.1 mmol/L, or in severe metabolic acidosis, consider haemodialysis.

Benzodiazepines
- Supportive therapy usually suffices.
- Consider oral activated charcoal if ingestion within 1 hour, provided they are not too drowsy.
- Flumazenil (a benzodiazepine antagonist) is only indicated for rare, life-threatening overdoses, i.e. respiratory depression or respiratory arrest.

Beta blockers
- Give IV atropine for hypotension and bradycardia.
- If this fails, give IV glucagon (to achieve a positive inotropic effect).
- Sometimes temporary pacing may be required if above measures fail.

Carbon monoxide
- Give 100% oxygen.
- Measure carboxyhaemoglobin levels to guide treatment.
- Consider giving hyperbaric oxygen if carboxyhaemoglobin levels >20%, patient is pregnant, neurological symptoms present, or cardiac dysrhythmias occur.

Cyanide
- Give IV dicobalt edetate; sodium nitrite followed by sodium thiosulphate are alternatives if dicobalt edetate not available.

- IV hydroxocobalamin can be used in the treatment of cyanide inhalation.

Digoxin
- Give oral activated charcoal if within 1 hour of ingestion.
- Correct any potassium disturbance and treat dysrhythmias with antiarrhythmic drugs (i.e. amiodarone, lidocaine).
- Give digoxin-specific antibody in serious overdose.
- If digoxin-specific antibody not available, provide supportive treatment for dysrhythmias using a combination of antiarrhythmic drugs, overdrive pacing and DC shock.

Iron
- Perform gastric lavage if within 1 hour of ingestion or if abdominal X-ray reveals tablets in the stomach.
- Give IV or IM desferrioxamine (an iron-chelating agent) depending on serum iron levels and clinical state.
- In severe iron overdose not responding to chelation therapy, haemodialysis is indicated.

Lithium
- Increase fluid intake orally or IV to increase urine production and elimination of drug.
- Provide supportive treatment.
- Sometimes whole bowel irrigation is considered to decrease absorption of lithium.
- In serious overdose arrange haemodialysis.

Opiates
- Give IV or IM naloxone (a short-acting opioid antagonist) in coma or respiratory depression.
- Owing to the short half-life of naloxone, patients should be observed after administration; in some cases repeated doses or an infusion may be required.

Organophosphates (insecticides, nerve gases)
- Wash contaminated skin and remove soiled clothing.
- Give atropine (IV or IM) to antagonize the effects of acetylcholine, which are intensified by organophosphates.
- Pralidoxime mesilate can be used as adjunct treatment (further reduces the effects of acetylcholine).

Paracetamol
- Liver damage can occur if more than 10 g of paracetamol is taken within 24 hours. In patients with certain risk factors, doses more than 5 g can cause liver damage.
- High-risk patients:
  - Long-term treatment with enzyme-inducing agents, e.g. rifampicin, carbamazepine, St John's wort.
  - Regularly consume alcohol in excess of recommended amounts.

- Likely to be glutathione depleted, e.g. eating disorder, starvation, HIV.
- Give activated charcoal if ingestion within 1 hour.
- Measure plasma paracetamol levels (if at least 4 hours have elapsed since ingestion) and plot on nomogram to decide if antidote required.
- If levels are in toxic range, give IV N-acetylcysteine infusion (if within 24 hours of ingestion – most effective if given within 8 hours of ingestion) or, alternatively, give oral methionine provided not vomiting (if within 10–12 hours of ingestion).
- Monitor LFTs, INR, U&Es and arterial blood gases.
- If there is doubt about amount or timing of the overdose the patient should be treated with the antidote.
- If there is continued deterioration (i.e. encephalopathy, rising INR, renal failure, metabolic acidosis), contact local liver unit as liver transplantation may need to be considered.

Theophylline
- Perform gastric lavage or give activated charcoal (only within 2 hours of ingestion).
- Give repeated activated charcoal 4-hourly until clinical condition improves or until charcoal appears in faeces.
- Correct any hypokalaemia with IV potassium chloride.
- Cardiac monitoring is required (as there is a danger of cardiac dysrhythmias).
- Give IV diazepam or lorazepam for any associated convulsions.
- Note: tachycardia, hyperglycaemia and hypokalaemia may be reversed with IV propranolol (contraindicated in asthmatics).

Tricyclic antidepressants (TCAs)
- Give oral activated charcoal 4-hourly until clinical condition improves.
- Attach cardiac monitor and monitor acid–base status.
- Treat any associated complications (e.g. convulsions, cardiac dysrhythmias).
- Acidosis should be corrected with IV sodium bicarbonate.
- Dysrhythmias usually settle with correction of hypoxia and acidosis.

CANCER THERAPY

Management guidelines

AIMS OF TREATMENT

- There are many chemotherapy agents used in clinical practice and with ongoing research new drugs are always in the pipeline. Most drugs can be used in the treatment of more than one type of cancer. Chemotherapy can be:
  - *Curative.*
  - *Neo-adjuvant:* initial chemotherapy given to shrink the primary tumour to facilitate surgery and/or radiotherapy.
  - *Adjuvant:* chemotherapy given after surgery and/or radiotherapy to prevent subclinical metastatic disease.
  - *Palliative:* to prolong life and palliate symptoms.
- There are many adverse effects that are common to most chemotherapy drugs; these are outlined below but each drug also has its own particular side-effects, e.g. doxorubicin is cardiotoxic.
- Common side-effects of chemotherapy agents:
  - Bone marrow suppression; causing anaemia, thrombocytopenia and neutropenia (neutropenic sepsis).
  - Alopecia.
  - Oral mucositis.
  - Tumour lysis syndrome.
  - Hyperuricaemia.
  - Nausea and vomiting.
  - Impaired fertility.
  - Thromboembolism.

CHEMOTHERAPY DRUGS

- Chemotherapy drugs can be divided into different types.

The Hands–on Guide to Clinical Pharmacology, 3rd Edition. By S Chatu.
Published 2010 by Blackwell Publishing Ltd.

Alkylating agents
* These drugs alter the DNA in cells and inhibit DNA synthesis. They attach alkyl groups to DNA bases which leads to:
    * Fragmentation of DNA by repair enzymes in their attempt to replace the alkyl groups.
    * Cross-linking of DNA, which prevents DNA from being separated for synthesis and transcription,
    * Cell mutation by causing mispairing of DNA.
* These agents are used in the treatment of solid tumours and leukaemia. Below is a list of alkylating agents:
    * Busulfan.
    * Carmustine.
    * Chlorambucil.
    * Cyclophosphamide.
    * Estramustine.
    * Ifosfamide.
    * Lomustine.
    * Melphalan.
    * Mitomycin C.
    * Thiotepa.
    * Treosulfan.

Antimetabolites
* These are structural analogues of naturally occurring metabolites that inhibit metabolism of compounds required for DNA, RNA and protein synthesis. There are three types.

Folic acid antagonists
* Inhibits dihydrofolate reductase, an enzyme involved in the formation of nucleotides required for DNA synthesis. An example is *methotrexate*, which is used in the treatment of solid tumours and haematological malignancies.

Pyrimidine antagonists
* Block synthesis of pyrimidine-containing nucleotides in DNA and RNA. They may also be incorporated into the DNA chain and terminate formation.
* Used in various types of cancer and examples include: *capecitabine, cytarabine, 5-fluorouracil (5-FU), gemcitabine.*

Purine antagonists
* Purines (adenine and guanine) are used to build the nucleotides of RNA and DNA. These agents inhibit production of purines and further inhibit DNA synthesis by becoming incorporated into the DNA molecule.
* Used in the treatment of leukaemia and commonly used agents are 6-mercaptopurine and fludarabine.

Antitubulin agents
* Bind to tubulin and inhibit microtubule formation, thereby impairing cell division. The vinca alkaloids are used in the treatment of haematological and solid tumours, whereas taxanes are only used in solid tumours.

- *Vinca alkaloids:*
  - Vinblastine.
  - Vincristine.
  - Vindesine.
  - Vinorelbine.
- *Taxanes:*
  - Docetaxel.
  - Paclitaxel.

Intercalating agents

- These agents become incorporated between bases along the DNA strand, changing the structure. This leads to prevention of DNA synthesis, induction of mutations and inhibition of transcription.
- *Platinum compounds*:
  - Carboplatin.
  - Cisplatin.
  - Oxaliplatin.
- *Anthracyclines*:
  - Bleomycin.
  - Dactinomycin.
  - Daunorubicin.
  - Doxorubicin.
  - Epirubicin.
  - Idarubicin.
  - Mitomycin.

Topoisomerase inhibitors

- These agents inhibit topoisomerase enzymes, which are involved in the coiling or uncoiling of DNA during replication. Used in the treatment of solid tumours, e.g. colorectal, ovarian and lung cancer:
  - Etoposide.
  - Irinotecan.
  - Topotecan.

New generation drugs
Monoclonal antibodies (MAbs)

- Immune human lymphoid cells are hybridized with cultured malignant murine plasma cells *in vitro*. These hybrids grow, and grow antibodies with a single defined specificity which may be cloned – MAbs. MAbs against tumour antigens can bind their specific targets and mediate lysis of tumour cells either through complement-mediated lysis or antibody-dependent cellular toxicity (e.g. CD20, CD52, human leukocyte antigen [HLA], etc).
- Current MAbs in use include:
  - *Bevacizumab*: colorectal cancer.
  - *Cetuximab*: colorectal cancer, head and neck cancer.
  - *Panitumumab*: colorectal cancer.
  - *Rituximab*: non-Hodgkin's lymphoma.
  - *Traztuzumab*: breast cancer.
- Common side-effects include allergic reaction (remember rodent component, therefore recognized as foreign body), rash, sore mouth, fatigue, nausea. Individual MAbs have their own specific side-effect profile.

Tyrosine kinase Inhibitors (TKIs)

* Tyrosine kinases are a family of proteins that are involved in cell signalling and have been implicated in the pathophysiology of cancer. Anticancer drug development has recently taken aim at these receptors. Small-molecule TKIs are a group of orally available compounds that selectively target and inhibit receptor tyrosine kinases (RTKs) and non-receptor tyrosine kinases (NRTKs).
* Current agents in clinical use:
    * *Erlotinib*: non-small cell lung cancer, pancreatic (in conjunction with gemcitabine).
    * *Gefitinib*: non-small cell lung cancer.
    * *Imatinib*: chronic lymphoid leukaemia (CLL), GIST.
    * *Lapatinib*: breast cancer (in conjunction with capecitabine).
    * *Sunitinib*: renal cell carcinoma, GI stromal tumour (GIST) (when refractory to imatinib).
* Commonest side-effects are rash and diarrhoea. Can also get neutropenia and hepatotoxicity, and a range of other less common side-effects.

INDEX

The Hands-on Guide to Clinical Pharmacology, 3rd Edition. By S Chatu.
Published 2010 by Blackwell Publishing Ltd.

Index compiled by Terry Halliday